Pregnancy After Loss

Also by Zoë Clark-Coates:

The Baby Loss Guide
Beyond Goodbye

Pregnancy After Loss

A day-by-day plan to reassure
and comfort you

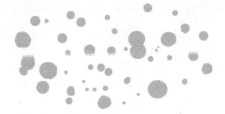

ZOË CLARK-COATES

First published in Great Britain in 2020 by Orion Spring
an imprint of The Orion Publishing Group Ltd
Carmelite House, 50 Victoria Embankment
London EC4Y 0DZ

An Hachette UK Company

1 3 5 7 9 10 8 6 4 2

Every effort has been made to ensure that the information in the
book is accurate. The information in this book may not be applicable
in each individual case so it is advised that professional medical advice is
obtained for specific health matters and before changing any medication or
dosage. Neither the publisher nor author accepts any legal responsibility
for any personal injury or other damage or loss arising from the use of
the information in this book. In addition, if you are concerned about
your diet or exercise regime and wish to change them, you should
consult a health practitioner first.

A CIP catalogue record for this book is
available from the British Library.

ISBN (Hardback) 978 1 4091 9594 8
ISBN (eBook) 978 1 4091 9595 5

Printed in Great Britain by Clays Ltd

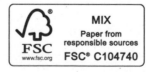

www.orionbooks.co.uk

Contents

PART 2: SUPPORT AND JOURNALLING

Introduction

We have come away for me to write. It's rare for me to have dedicated time to sit and pour out my heart onto the page, and we have found the best chance of creating this space is to leave the country. So here I am, sitting at a desk in front of a window, looking out onto white sand and palm trees. The sun should be shining, and I should be able to hear children playing happily in the pool below, but a tropical storm hit five days ago, and it has still got a firm hold on this part of the coast. So instead of gentle waves lapping at the shore, I am watching mega waves which are delighting only the most experienced surfers. Red flags pepper the sand, warning of imminent danger and alerting people to the risk they're taking should they enter the water.

The fact that this scene is a metaphor for pregnancy after loss hasn't escaped me. One starts a new pregnancy like one would start a vacation – full of high expectations, the excitement of feeling the sun on your skin, the anticipation of peace and relaxation, and a hope that the biggest worry for the next week will be which cocktail you should order. But sadly this isn't always how it goes. And if your holiday is spoiled once, that experience is likely to change how you view future trips. Similarly, pregnancy post-loss is very different from pregnancy pre-loss. Once you have encountered the heart-shattering experience of losing a child (however early or late in pregnancy the loss was, or loss post-birth) the terrain of subsequent pregnancies changes forever. Instead of waking up each morning expecting to sit in the sun, you are instead nervously peering through the curtains, dreading the sight of rain. Where you may have once happily strolled into the sea for a swim, you are now too scared of the creatures that you know inhabit the water, which you would have previously never even considered. Your world has changed forever. Your eyes have been opened and, for many people, this means fear has stopped being an imaginary monster under the bed, and become instead a real-life beast interfering in every part of your life.

If you are nodding right now and saying, 'YES, this is me', let me assure you of this – you don't have to dread the next nine months, and you don't need to fast-forward time. I promise you can enjoy this pregnancy. You can use this period of time to gain strength, learn new skills, process more grief layers (if you feel you need to do this) and enjoy growing your child within.

That said, I can't promise you this road will be easy; I can't tell you that you won't need to battle fear, as you may need to use your sword, my sword, and others' swords to fight back the terror that will want to take up residence in your heart and mind. There may also be many occasions where you need to search for your Wonder Woman pants (always my superhero of choice) in order to deal with things you would rather not face, ask the questions you would rather not ask, and go to places you would prefer not to enter, such as hospitals and doctors' waiting rooms. But I promise you do have the strength to take on anything that comes your way. How do I know this? Because you have survived a loss already, and that makes you strong. You have survived one of the worst things that could ever happen to a human, and you have emerged on the other side. So you can do this too. And I will do this with you.

I want to say this to you, and I need you to hear it. It is okay to feel scared. It is understandable that you are terrified. You shouldn't feel any shame for experiencing any feeling. Society may tell you that you should just feel gratitude for being pregnant, and that may make you feel awful for battling a host of other emotions, but it is 100 per cent natural to feel the way you do, and I hope my words in this book can reassure you of that.

After my own losses, I needed someone to walk alongside me in pregnancy, to remind me I had the strength to fight the good fight, and it is my privilege to do that for you. I needed someone to help me silence the torment in my mind that constantly whispered in my ear that things may not end well, and I will try to do this for you. I feel I have learnt a valuable secret, and this is it – the best way to get through pregnancy post-loss is to try to presume all is well. You have to have blinkers on: horses wear blinkers to shield their eyes so things approaching in their blind spots can't spook them; it means they can only see the path directly in front of them, and this is what you need to try to do. Your key to enjoying this period of time, and feeling able to make it through, is by holding on to the belief that you will end up with a baby in your arms. I understand that this is incredibly hard when you have had previous tragedy to deal with (everyone who has lived this understands that it is a mighty task), but I hope my words will help you to know you are wholly equipped for this battle, you do have the strength, and I will be cheering you on along the way.

You can do this, my friend!

We can do it together.

Love,

Zoë

xxxx

My Story in Brief

Having seen a close friend go through the horrendous experience of miscarriage and stillbirth, I had put off having children, as I didn't know if I could personally cope with the possibility of such a loss. However, having been married for over 12 years to my soulmate (we married young) and setting up a successful business, suddenly my biological clock started ticking. Yes, I too thought this was an urban myth, that one day you could be satisfied with no children, then the next you have a burning desire to reproduce, but it happened to me; I can confirm it is real.

After a while, I knew I was pregnant, but, heartbreakingly, it ended in a miscarriage, and my way of coping was almost to pretend it hadn't happened. I didn't want to be one of those statistics, which state that up to one in four pregnancies ends in miscarriage. Surely if I didn't acknowledge it, it didn't happen? I pushed all emotion down, and we went into total denial. We later named this baby Cobi.

Within a couple of months, we were blessed to get pregnant again. We decided to keep it a secret from the family and tell them as a surprise at Christmas.

We went for our first scan, and there was a heart-stopping moment when the sonographer said: 'Are you sure you have your dates right? I can't see anything.' Following our assurance that the dates were indeed correct, she suddenly announced, 'Oh, there it is', and on the screen, we witnessed the miracle of life, our tiny baby, wriggling around, with its little heartbeat fluttering away. We were, of course, over the moon. The sonographer mentioned that she could see a pool of blood in the womb, and warned me I should expect a little blood loss at some point, but not to worry about it at all. That evening I did get a little spotting, and if I'm honest I did panic. I think any woman will agree that if you see any signs of blood while pregnant, fear swells from nowhere. But by the following day the spotting had stopped, so peace returned.

A while later, I caught the flu and was bedridden for a week. Then, as quickly as it had stopped, the bleeding started again, but this time it felt different. We found a clinic who agreed to scan me. After what felt like an age, we were called into the scanning room, and the doctor immediately activated the all-telling machine. There on the screen, we saw our baby for the second time – kicking away, showing no signs of distress or concern . . . what a relief!

We were due to go to a party on Saturday evening, so hoping that resting might stop any further bleeding I stayed in bed, continually doing that maternal stroke of the stomach, which somehow feels like you're comforting and caring for your child within. But when I got up that evening, I felt a sudden rush of blood, and I knew my baby had just died. I lay on the floor begging God to save her, crying out to the only One who truly controls life and death, but I knew it was in vain. Deep down I knew she was destined to be born into heaven, not onto the earth. Mother's instinct? Who knows, but I knew her little heart was no longer beating within her or me.

We rushed to hospital where I was sadly met with little concern; I was even asked if it was an IVF baby as I was so upset. 'Why?' I asked. 'Is it not normal to cry over a naturally conceived child?' They had no answer. They didn't examine me; I was just told, 'There is nothing we can do. Let nature take its course. What will be, will be.' I was given an appointment for an emergency scan in a week and told to go home to bed.

The next day, a Sunday, the bleeding slowed down, and

we left messages on numerous clinic answering machines begging for an appointment as soon as possible. The following morning, before 9am, we got a call from a wonderful clinic telling us to come over, and they would scan me. That was to be one of the longest journeys of my life.

We were called from the waiting area, and into a small room. I was told to get on the bed, and the scanner was booted up. After what seemed like an eternity of silence, I finally willed up the courage to ask, 'Can you see the baby? Is everything OK?' I didn't need to ask, my baby was still; the only movement on the screen came from my body, not hers. My question was met with the worst answer: 'Zoë, I'm sorry to say there isn't a heartbeat.' I screamed. I pleaded for a second scan, which she did. She then went to get a consultant; he came in, shaking his head, saying the same words, ones that would become very familiar to us over the coming months: 'I'm so sorry.'

We were quickly put in a tiny room, where we sobbed, wailed, and clung to each other; we called our family, and hearing the words coming out of our mouths, the nightmare of our reality dawned on us: our baby had died. She was still here with us, but we would never hold her hand, or rock her to sleep. 'What now?' we asked. We were told we could go the surgical route or the natural route. I chose the natural path, as the thought of going to a hospital where my baby would be just extracted from me seemed wrong; she was my baby, and I wanted to keep her with me for as long as possible.

What I wasn't prepared for was that the ordeal would go on for a week. A scan after a few days showed the baby had developed further, which is apparently totally normal, as the blood supply is still making the baby grow. However, her heart remained still, no spark of life was seen. I heard them say, 'No, Zoë, sadly your baby hasn't miraculously come back to life. Yes, we know you had hoped it would happen.'

Was I wrong to hope this might be the case? What if I prayed non-stop? What if I kept rubbing my stomach night and day? Would her heart start to beat again? I had been told by a nurse that there was one case of this happening somewhere in the world once. So was I misguided to believe I could be the second?

We returned home, and the days passed, long and slow. Someone asked me how I could allow a dead baby to stay inside me. 'Because it's my baby,' I said. Why one would presume that her death made her any less precious, or me any less loving, I'm not sure. For some, carrying a dead baby within seems creepy, morbid and wrong, but to me I was being her mother, keeping her safe in the place that had become her haven. I felt she was entitled to remain there until she decided to leave, it wasn't my place to suddenly evict her, and I was prepared to wait as long as it needed for her to dictate the timing of our meeting.

A week to the day after her heartbeat stopped, labour started, and within 24 hours, I had delivered my child: my daughter, Darcey.

For the next six weeks, my body raged with pregnancy hormones as it wrongly believed I was still carrying a child. Sickness continued, day and night, along with indigestion and headaches. What had once been reassuring symbols of pregnancy were now distressing reminders of what was no more. The oddest thing then started to occur: almost daily, strangers would randomly ask me if I had children. Each time, it was like I was being thumped in the stomach. I instantly faced the dilemma of whether to protect the feelings of the person who had just asked me this very innocent question. Did I say, 'No, I haven't'? By doing so, I felt I would be denying my child's existence. Or should I bravely say, 'I have actually, but they died.' I tried both, and both felt wrong, and I quickly learnt I was in a lose-lose situation, and I should do whatever felt right at the time.

I was met with lots of well-meaning statements like, 'At least it proves you can conceive,' and, 'Sometimes the womb just needs practice.' Thankfully the less sensitive comments were a minority, and I was blessed to have my husband – my hero – by my side. He may not have always known what to say, but he was wise enough to know that words often aren't needed and that just to hold me would frequently be enough. And then there were my parents, who sat with us and filled endless buckets with their tears while helping to empty ours. The rest of our family and friends were fantastic, their support was tangible, and though most had no comprehension of what we were experiencing, they made it clear to us that they were there, and that meant the world to us.

Some might think that these experiences would extinguish the biological clock, but they didn't. They only increased my desire to have a baby, but the simultaneous fear that I would never become a mum to a living child was overwhelming.

Two months later, I tragically lost my third baby (Bailey) via a miscarriage. We kept this to ourselves, as we felt the family had gone through enough. They were under the assumption we had only ever lost one baby, and to tell them about this loss would mean admitting to them, and to ourselves, that this was our third child to grace the heavenly gates.

Then we got pregnant again, and I am sure you can imagine the terror we felt. I found it hard to believe that this pregnancy would end up any differently to the first three; after all, I had no positive experience to cling to. Due to my medical history, my pregnancy was monitored closely by a consultant, and this meant I got fortnightly scans. In the week leading up to each scan, I would be gripped by nerves and would have to practise relaxation exercises to cope with the stress. As the scan was happening, while I could actually see my baby on the screen, I would feel a rare sense of peace. How I wished I could stay right there in that room, watching my little one grow, so I knew she was safe and well. The peace that the scan brought would last a couple of hours, and then that niggling fear would return, as just because my baby was OK earlier didn't mean she was OK now. I guess to someone who has never experienced pregnancy loss, this may seem a crazy way to think, but if you have been there, you will understand this mindset and empathise.

But this time was different as, after nine very long months, we were finally handed our beautiful daughter, Esmé Emilia Promise. She was delivered by C-section, weighing 6lb 15oz. The relief was profound, and there are no words to explain the happiness of finally getting to hold and protect my tiny little girl.

We loved being parents so much; the thought of having another child was mentioned when she was 18 months old, even though we had declared to everyone we knew that we would be stopping at one! Nothing had prepared us for the amount of joy a little one can add to your life. There was nothing about being a mum I didn't love, so we decided to try for a brother or sister for Esmé.

Naïvely, having borne a healthy, thriving child who went to full term, we believed our dealings with miscarriage and loss were in the past, and any further pregnancies would follow the course of our last one, rather than our first three. We were wrong.

We got pregnant, and all the initial scans were perfect. Then at one of our appointments, the scan showed our baby's heartbeat had stopped. Time went into slow motion when we were told; I literally couldn't speak. Nothing had prepared me to tumble through that hidden trap door, from expectant mother to missed miscarriage, a fourth time. I misguidedly thought that to lose a child when you already have one would hurt less, but I was wrong; it is different but not less. You aren't grieving the fact that you may never be a mother to a living child (as you are already), but it hurts in a lot of new ways. We were constantly asking ourselves, would this baby have laughed in the same way as our little girl? Would he have talked in the same way? The grief was consuming, and I felt like I had been pushed off a cliff edge with no warning. We named our baby Samuel.

In a bid to try to protect our little girl from seeing any

upset, I only allowed myself to cry in private and forced myself to keep things as normal as possible for her, but this was an Everest-type challenge, I'm not going to lie.

I opted to take the medical route this time, and within days I found myself in a hospital bed, filling in paperwork, sobbing after the nurse asked two questions: 'Would you like a postmortem, and would you like the remains back?' Can any mother ever be prepared to answer such questions?

In medical terms, those who die in utero within the first 24 weeks of life are known as 'retained products of conception', so perhaps you should expect to be asked these questions while filling in a form. I am one of millions, however, who feel you should not have to face them. I know for some people these aren't babies, they are just a group of cells, and I respect that this is their opinion; but to my husband and me, this was our child, not just a potential person, but an actual person, and he deserved to be acknowledged as such.

We were blessed to get pregnant for a sixth time and, after telling the family on Christmas Eve, I went upstairs to find I had started to bleed. The bleeding continued for days, and when I finally managed to speak to a GP, I was told I had definitely miscarried, and there was no need for a scan. That crushing sadness overtook me again, and those who have experienced this first-hand will know you literally have to remind yourself to breathe. Human functions seem to disappear, and you feel you're free-falling over a ravine. I held on to the knowledge that to have my daughter should, of course, be enough. If we were never blessed with another child, we were one of the lucky couples who at least had the opportunity to raise one little girl. So we painted a smile on our faces and tried to give our daughter a fantastic Christmas.

However, by 5 January, I was feeling so ill I decided to go for a scan, in case I needed another operation, and to our surprise, they could still see a baby, and all looked OK. I was told that this by no means meant all would be fine, but it was a good sign, and I should book another scan in a couple of weeks. During this time, my sickness increased, and by the time I went for my next scan, I was sicker than I had ever been while pregnant. The scan commenced, and the doctor announced he could see two little lives on the screen. 'Yes, Zoë, you are having twins . . .' Cue Andy and me staring at him in shock and excitement in equal measure. He did warn us that one of the twins looked more developed than the other, and that was not a good sign. With that information in mind, we were prepared (as prepared as one can ever be, that is) that we might not end this pregnancy journey with two healthy babies in our arms, but we prayed that we would.

Tragically we did indeed go on to lose one of our precious babies, and we named her Isabella. Our other twin hung on, and we felt blessed to have one baby growing safely within, but heartbroken for the baby we lost.

What followed was a minefield of a pregnancy. I had to have my gallbladder removed; I had liver problems, placenta previa, symphysis pubis dysfunction (SPD), and my placenta was stuck to the old C-section scar. The final blow came when I developed obstetric cholestasis, an intense itching of the skin, but our little warrior braved it all! When Brontë Jemima Hope finally appeared in all her glory in August 2011, she was declared a miracle baby, and I don't think we have stopped smiling since.

'Was it all worth it?' some may ask. Of course! 'Do you wish you had detonated your biological clock as it caused you so much pain?' Absolutely not. I have two wonderful little girls, whom I simply adore; they have made every single tear worth shedding. I'm so proud to be a mother, and I hope the trauma I have gone through makes me a better wife, mother and friend. My passion is to raise my girls now to love life and embrace every opportunity life hands to them.

What I have learnt through this heartbreak is that I believe every child matters, however far along the pregnancy. I also learnt a lot about grief. I was a trained counsellor before going through loss myself, but I quickly realised all the training in the world couldn't make you understand the first-hand experience of baby loss.

I learnt that everyone is entitled to grieve differently. Some may not even feel the need to shed a tear, some may sob endlessly, and both are fine. For the heartbroken, however, acknowledging the loss is essential and it's imperative to both physical health and mental well-being to grieve. Life may never be the same again when you have been to such depths of darkness, but we can move forward, with as little scar tissue on the soul as possible, and saying goodbye was the key for me.

Pregnancy after loss taught me first-hand the power of the mind. It also showed me fear could control and ruin anything, and I made a determined effort to battle it rather than succumb to it. I also learnt how to hold on to hope, and I think this was one of my biggest life lessons . . . Somewhere along the way (perhaps in childhood), I had decided to prepare myself for the worst in a bid to protect my heart if things went wrong. Pregnancy after loss showed me you can't prepare for heartache, and if you try to, you end up robbing yourself of joy. Additionally, the more you look at the negative, the harder the journey is to navigate. So I learnt to celebrate every milestone, and embrace each day. No, I couldn't say for sure my baby would be fine tomorrow, but I could rejoice that they were OK today.

I have written about my story in more detail in my previous books if you would like to read more about my journey through loss.

Pregnancy After Loss is the book that I needed in pregnancy. I needed words to reassure me, stories to make me feel less alone, and advice on how to navigate fear. I wanted to know I wasn't weird to feel how I was feeling and I wanted help to enjoy the journey through pregnancy. I hope this book is all of that and more for you.

PART 1

Why Is Pregnancy After Loss Different?

There are hundreds of pregnancy manuals in the shops, but few of them address what you need when you are facing a pregnancy after losing a child. What might be an exciting milestone to someone in their first pregnancy may be a frightening reminder to someone else about a time when things went wrong before. I know that when I was pregnant after my losses, I found little comfort – or relevance – in the standard advice. What I needed was a battle plan – a step-by-step guide to get from A to Z. Nine months feels like a lifetime when you are battling entirely justified worry and panic. I needed a book that acknowledged what I had previously gone through, and reassured me I wasn't crazy for feeling like I did, but then empowered me to move forwards. I needed to be shown skills, actions and tips not only to help me to survive, but just as importantly to help me to flourish. Within this book, I have tried to deliver the advice and understanding that I needed, which I learnt first-hand, and through working with thousands of people just like you. If you can commit to trusting me, we can walk this path together so that you feel less alone.

The second section of this book will address each day of your pregnancy. But before we get there, I want to offer some advice and techniques that may help you.

MANAGING ANXIETY AND FEAR

Anxiety can make us feel like we have a sense of control. We may feel that by obsessing over every eventuality we can somehow control the outcome and change our destiny; I think this is why we cling to the things we fear. The issue with this is we are creating platforms for terror to take up residence in our heads, and the more ground we offer to our fears, the less space we have for peace. Before we know it, the landscape in front of us is dominated by anguish, and it's only then that we can see anxiety has not given us more control, we have in fact handed over every little bit of our power to worry. We don't control our lives anymore; fear does. We are at its mercy, and we can go from being a fearless warrior to cowering in the corner of the room.

Fear is such a powerful emotion. We can even start to fear the fear itself. So even when we are not frightened about something, we are led to make choices that mean we only walk down safe paths, where anxiety won't haunt us. When I was considering whether I could face pregnancy again post-loss, I felt that there was no way I could handle it. I was terrified of the dread I believed would descend. This meant I was instantly allowing fear to control my life: I didn't just fear pregnancy; I was dreading the alarm that I may feel when pregnant. These emotions were all completely normal, and even rational, but that didn't mean I wanted the terror consume me, or that I had to accept it as my truth. I had to believe I had the power, as do you, to work at not letting worry control my future. By taking time to think and process, you can carefully consider what you would like your future to include. When I considered this, I decided I desperately wanted a baby to raise in my home. To allow this dream to become a reality, I needed to armour up and prepare to battle my trepidation; I had to resist allowing the fear of loss to shape my life choices. Facing the fear didn't mean I would automatically get my heart's desire (a baby in my arms), it just meant that I wasn't going to let my worry rob me of the chance of getting it.

When I was considering what to write on these pages, I knew there was one vital thing I needed to include, and it's a pledge I would ask you to make right now.

> **'I pledge not to use forums or the internet to investigate my concerns. I will speak to my health team if I have any worries.'**

Now I know for some of you this may be like asking you to give up your right arm. We live in a society where it's the norm to have access to an abundance of information 24/7. And you are, quite naturally, desperate for reassurance. However, when we google symptoms or concerns we are often absorbing a host of information that does not apply to us or our situation. In a bid to find peace, we discover more potential issues we didn't even know were a possibility, so we gain more fear. And if we do see some snippets of information that reassure us, we have no clue whether they are relevant to our situation or not; so this could be false reassurance, and in fact do us further harm. This is why the internet can be such a dangerous place when we are operating from a feeling of terror. No one on the planet shares your history or your future, and the same applies to your baby, so there is no point in comparing your story with chapters in other people's books. So please consider taking the pledge; let's shut the door to this easy point of access, which allows additional anxiety to enter.

The Mariposa Trust asked 224 people who had previously encountered loss about their experience of a subsequent pregnancy. Here are the results:

- 96.77% of people said they were scared during subsequent pregnancies, with 81.57% saying their fear lasted throughout the pregnancy.

When asked how quickly they tried for another child:

- 48.65% started trying within three months of losing a baby
- 22.07% started trying within six months of losing a baby
- 10.81% started trying within 9–12 months of losing a baby
- 18.47% started trying 12+ months after losing a baby

COPING WITH PANIC AND TERROR

When terror grips you, you may have no idea how you will survive the next minute, let alone the next day. Your heart starts to race, your temperature may soar, and you feel like you may faint.

Unless you have experienced a panic attack yourself, it is hard to comprehend their magnitude. People can even be taken to hospital convinced they are having a heart attack due to the severity of the symptoms. You may feel you can't breathe, or that you are dying. Panic attacks can control your life in two ways: firstly, when you are having an attack, you can be brought to your knees. Secondly, the dread of an attack creeping up without warning can make you feel on constant high alert.

Excitement, fear, nerves, upset, worry, trepidation – any of these feelings can activate your fight-or-flight response and trigger a panic attack. Once the cortisol is surging around your system, it can be hard to get it back under control, but it is possible to recreate the balance.

Let me reassure you it is possible to deactivate an extreme panic response and to get it to release its hold on you, but it will take time, work, and you may need help from a specialist such as a counsellor or your doctor. So let me say this to you and please hear it – if you feel desperate, please speak to your doctor or someone you trust and see if counselling may give you the freedom you long for. You deserve a good life, without panic being at the core of your thinking, and I promise you it is achievable.

While you are working towards a pregnancy and a life without crippling worry, let's address how you might manage the symptoms when they occur. I can't remove your stress, but I hope I can help you handle it. I want to give you as many tools as I can to help you navigate the fear and worry right now. Some of these tools may help you, others may not, but I will share everything that has helped me personally, and techniques I have taught to tens of thousands of people over the years. Imagine you have a backpack on your shoulders, and I am passing you tools to put in your bag. If and when you need a tool to navigate a tough path, I hope you can reach right in there and pull out something that may help you in your moment of need. So let's start filling your backpack!

Panic comes in lots of guises; it may be just a sense of impending doom, or a feeling like you are on a big-dipper ride, and your stomach keeps flipping. You may be able to determine easily what is causing these feelings (i.e. an upcoming appointment or scan), or it may come knocking on your door out of nowhere. The latter is probably the hardest to explain and cope with, as the sensation can feel utterly irrational when you are experiencing it, and, without an obvious reason, it is hard to explain and verbalise to yourself or others. The most common thing people say to me when they are experiencing this type of dread is, 'Am I going mad?' The answer 99 per cent of the time is, 'No, you are simply suffering from panic and anxiety.'

Panic attacks will manifest differently in every person, but they are often sudden, debilitating and paralysing. Often people will feel hot or cold; their heart will pound and they will feel overcome with emotion – upset, unease, agitation, distress. They may be able to confirm what triggered it (i.e. some people get panic attacks when entering a busy room, so their trigger is super-clear), or they may be unaware of what has caused the attack. One of the many issues with panic attacks is people don't only fear experiencing the panic attack itself; they worry they will encounter one, so they become hyper-alert. Whether they experience an attack or not, an occasion or even life can feel ruined.

So how do you navigate a panic attack? Firstly, we need to determine what has triggered it. Can you identify a triggering incident? If so, is it possible to avoid this situation? If your trigger, for instance, is busy bars, unless you are employed in one, it may be easier to avoid going to a bar until you have sought help. Avoidable triggers that don't really harm your life or shrink your world substantially are easier to cope with than unpredictable triggers, as even though the reaction is 100 per cent out of your control, you can consciously avoid the situation. So my first piece of advice is: try to identify your triggers and decide which are avoidable and which aren't.

While you are under considerable stress or worry, try to limit your exposure to triggers and spend as much time as possible practising relaxation techniques and doing things that bring you peace. Unavoidable triggers would be circumstances such as needing to go to see the doctor or midwife, or hospital appointments. These are necessary for your health, and that of your baby, so it is not possible to avoid these situations. In these cases, you will need to deal with the panic and symptoms as they happen.

When trepidation is building ahead of a specific trigger like a medical appointment, I have written a seven-day plan for the week leading up to the event. I urge you to be faithful and consistent in following this plan, as the key is being diligent in carrying out the exercises so you are well practised. That means when fear tries to take hold, you will have additional skills to control the symptoms.

Another key to living with underlying panic and worry is to try to change your feelings about your panic responses. I tried to see my pounding heart as excitement rather than fear; my fast breathing as anticipation rather than worry. Whenever I got that sinking feeling in my stomach, I told myself these feelings would encourage me to power on through, and make it to the other side. By changing my thought pattern surrounding the symptoms it almost de-empowered them from controlling me. Changing how you think doesn't happen overnight, and it's not easy . . . but it is possible with work and commitment.

I also want to encourage you to change how you view short-term stress. For most of us, we have been taught to view it as the enemy, and of course it may often be just that. However, at times it can also help us. Short-term stress can sometimes encourage us to move in the right direction, or radically change our route of travel. It can energise us and empower us to not give up. Surprisingly it can even boost our immune system. It can make us divert from dangerous situations into a place of safety. It can make us reach for our dreams (even if that comes at a cost): these are all ways stress can positively influence us.

In recent years several medical studies have been carried out on the value of stress and the function of it in our lives. One of the more surprising findings was how the neurohormone oxytocin plays a vital role in how we respond. Most people are unaware that oxytocin is released when we are stressed, as it's often purely linked with love and intimacy, but it is actually a stress hormone. When the hormone is released it makes us crave intimacy and encourages us to connect with people at a deeper level. It can also make us more compassionate and caring. This means when we are under stress we can actually become more responsive and empathetic. Stress can make us strive to share more, care more and build valuable relationships with those around us. I believe this is why we form such strong bonds with people who are walking on similar paths to ourselves. When we are simultaneously feeling anxious we can empathise, but perhaps more importantly we *want* to empathise, as oxytocin makes us want to draw closer to people. So you see, short-term stress isn't always a bad thing – it can have huge benefits too.

7-DAY PLAN AHEAD OF A TRIGGERING EVENT

DAY 1

Spend six minutes today practising relaxation exercises (find these on page 30). Three times today, take two minutes to learn how to focus on taking deep breaths. When we are stressed, our breathing can be shallow. When we are relaxed, our breathing becomes deep and even. You can help your body to feel relaxed by consciously sending deep breaths into your abdomen and focusing on the sensation of the breath, instead of on your racing thoughts.

If you would like to be guided through these exercises and hear relaxing music head to https://www.thewaitingroom.life/

Bonus tip

Do you have a hobby? If not, I recommend finding one, as it is a great distraction in stressful times. Maybe it is time to take up a new craft or skill? Perhaps you could learn a new language? Maybe you could work towards a new qualification? There is no better time to learn something new than when you are going through a period of time that's exacerbating nerves, so I encourage you to think hard about taking up a new project. Make it something you love, so that you look forward to it, rather than seeing it as a chore.

One thing that helped me cope with pregnancy post-loss was sudoku. I hate maths, so I have no clue what made me choose this, probably because I could do it from bed or wherever I was, but I promise you it helped me so much. When I was focusing on those puzzles, my brain had no room to venture off into dark places; try to find your equivalent.

DAY 2

Spend nine minutes today practising relaxation exercises. Ideally, divide this time into three lots of three minutes: practise once on waking, once mid-afternoon and once before bed.

If your heart starts pounding at any point today, try to tell yourself this is due to excitement, and it is nothing to fear. Put your hand on your chest, and feel each one of those beats. Every time you feel a beat either say out loud, or in your mind: 'Thank you for beating. Thank you for keeping me alive. Thank you for pumping blood around my body and keeping me and my baby alive.' Just taking the time to breathe deeply, feel gratitude, and not allowing the physical symptoms to bring panic to your mind, should make your heart rate return to normal.

Bonus tip

Try to do something to treat yourself today – maybe that's a long soak in the bath? Maybe it's applying a face mask, or perhaps it's eating a food you love? Just do something that makes you feel spoilt and something that brings you joy. Plus, take time to do your new hobby, or to think about what you might take up.

DAY 3

Spend 10 minutes today practising relaxation exercises. Ideally, do five minutes in the morning and five minutes in the evening. Write down how you are feeling and allow yourself to cry, laugh, or process things you are concerned over.

Bonus tip

Try to spend time with people you love and connect with them on a deep level. When we feel stressed, oxytocin is released and this makes us want to be around those who make us feel understood and cared for. I encourage you to listen to this internal desire, as human connection changes everyday experiences. This hormone is actually kind of magical: did you know that one of its main roles in the body is to protect our cardiovascular system from the trauma of stress? And this may blow your mind . . . one of its hero tasks is to protect the heart. The heart has receptors for oxytocin, and it helps heart cells regenerate and heal from trauma damage; how amazing is that! So the saying 'love can help us heal' is clinically correct. Spend as much time as you can with the people you love . . . it will help you navigate stressful days.

DAY 4

Throughout today, spend at least 15 minutes practising your relaxation exercises. I encourage you to divide it into three lots of five minutes – once on waking, once in the afternoon and once before bed.

Bonus tip

During the day, find a piece of music that makes you feel happy and relaxed – listen to it and, if you feel able to, have a dance (even if you only imagine yourself dancing).

DAY 5

Over the course of the day spend 20 minutes practising your relaxation exercises. Perhaps break it down to four lots of five minutes and set an alarm to ensure you complete the task. If you can spend longer, then do. The more the better.

As you are approaching the appointment or event you are concerned about, it is totally natural to experience physical responses to stress. Most people say their heart pounds and their stomach feels like it is on a big-dipper ride. Both of these are classic responses to stress. If you experience them try to tell yourself that these are also common responses to excitement. So instead of thinking, 'I'm terrified' when your heart pounds, change that internal dialogue to, 'I'm excited that this will soon be done.' Simple changes to thought processes can be highly effective over the long term in reducing the symptoms.

Bonus tip

Try to have one meaningful conversation with someone about how you feel. Sharing your worries can be so helpful. Make time to do your new hobby.

DAY 6

Now we are getting closer to the date of your triggering event. This is often when panic may go up a notch, and you may start feeling more overwhelmed. You will need to practise relaxation exercises more, and use distraction as much as possible. I suggest a minimum of 30 minutes of relaxation practice today, ideally divided into two lots of 15 minutes.

Bonus tip

In addition to practising relaxation techniques, I recommend that you find a book that captivates your attention and/or watch films or TV shows that entertain you and keep you focused. Try to ensure these are not related to pregnancy or childbirth, or anything that might trigger more worry, or make your adrenaline flow. You are looking for escapism here, but want to stay calm.

I know you probably wish you could fast-forward time! Believe me, I get that. I must have said it and felt it myself a million times. Even though you can't fast-forward 24 hours at will, you can make time feel like it's going faster or slower by what you do with it.

Think of the activities that make time pass more quickly for you. Art, cooking, reading, walking, craft? Try to take time for hobbies and tasks that use up time and keep your mind occupied.

DAY 7

Start your day with five minutes of relaxation exercises.

The day of the appointment. Remind yourself that you can and will handle this. If you feel the anxiety rising, return to your deep breathing exercises.

- Say to yourself: I was born for this moment. I have the strength to get through this and survive it.
- If fear starts shouting in your ear, 'What if this happens, or what if this or that is said?' try to ignore the chatter. Remind yourself that right now all is well. You are only tasked with surviving this minute; you can't influence the future by worrying about it.
- Keep refocusing your attention on the now. Whatever task you need to do, such as having a shower or drying your hair, I suggest you totally focus on that task. If your thoughts drift to your fears, (and they probably will), gently bring your mind back to the present and think about the task at hand.
- If you have time to fill in the day, do your hobby or another task and keep focused on it. When the time

comes to leave for your appointment the same strategy applies: only focus on the journey itself, nothing beyond that. You tackle the task a step at a time, always staying present in that moment, focusing on your deep breathing.

- Some people find comfort in holding an item in their hand. I found a beautifully smooth pebble and kept it in my pocket. Whenever I was nervous I would hold it and rub it with my fingers. I would focus my mind on how soft it was, the shape it was, the journey it had travelled. This really helped me when I was trying to stay present.

Conclude your day with five minutes of relaxation exercises. While doing them repeat the words, 'I made it through today, I did well.'

WHEN FEAR DESCENDS OUT OF NOWHERE

If fear has gripped you, how do you navigate it? The first step is to try to determine what has caused it, in a bid to either deal with the trigger or avoid the trigger in the future, and cope with the symptoms.

When you're in the throes of panic, you need to try to make yourself feel secure, and this will look different for every person. For some, security means heading to the beach and the outdoors; for others it may be just hiding away in their bedroom – only you know where you feel safest.

Some will need to talk about their concerns – those that are valid/rational or those that are irrational (though of course irrational worries will feel totally rational at the point that you are feeling them). A conversation won't help everyone – some will need silence, or perhaps distraction by listening to music or watching a film. The aim is to calm your pulse rate and to regain a sense of composure. Sometimes breathing in and out of a paper bag can help calm your pulse rate, so it is worth having one to hand.

Knowing a fear or panic attack could strike at any point is so scary, but on the flip side, they can vanish without warning too. I hear so many stories from people who just woke up one morning and all worry had vanished, even after being tortured by it for years, so I hope this brings you hope. Fear can leave as quickly as it arrives.

People experience fear or panic attacks for a wide variety of reasons – some are due to trauma and the fight-or-flight response becoming almost permanently engaged; some are as a result of mental health conditions such as depression and general anxiety disorders or post-traumatic stress disorder, which is very common following losing a baby. Some are due to physical illness, grief or other life crises. Some are purely down to chemical or hormonal swings. Often people never investigate their fear or panic triggers; they are just mightily relieved when they end.

Another reason extreme anxiety can take hold is if people don't actually know how they feel or why they feel the way they do about something. (The something may be a situation, an experience, a relationship, a trauma, an emotion etc.) The reason people don't know is because they rarely give themselves time to process, analyse or digest emotions, feelings and circumstances. This is why talking can truly unlock people who are gripped by anxious thoughts; once they have ascertained what they feel or think or believe or fear, the panic gradually lifts off them.

An important question I often get asked by people who are struggling with anxiety is: 'How do I stay present and in the moment when I have to make lots of decisions and choices about the future?' Well, this is tough, especially if the situations you are considering induce panic. My first piece of advice would be to try to empower those around you to make any small decisions for you, whether this is about general life stuff, such as what's for supper or where do we visit today.

Releasing this control can be hard for some people, especially if they like to be in control of everything and anything, but for others, it will make life a little simpler on a day-to-day basis.

When you know a bigger decision needs to be made, and it can't be delegated to another person, give yourself space to think and time to process any feelings that are generated. Tell those around you how they can best support you (if you even know, as sometimes it is hard to know what you want when you feel overwhelmed). Perhaps talking with someone would help you? Maybe you need silence or time alone to calmly consider your choices? Try to look rationally at the decision at hand, weigh up both sides and then ask yourself this big question – 'If I had no anxiety, is this the decision I would be making?'

I'm not suggesting you will entirely overcome all worry – as it may sadly just be part of your life right now – but just consider the consequences of letting fear be the dominant voice in your head. Let me give you an example. When thinking about trying again for a baby, I was so nervous. Fear was bellowing in my ears, 'Don't do it, you will just go through loss again.' For a while, I wasn't ready to try again, but after a time I was ready, despite being scared. At that point the dread of not having more children was stronger than the qualm of going through more loss. So, to be clear, at no point was I free of fear, I just had to choose what was best for my family and me. For some, the horror of loss is enough to make them believe it's best not to try for more babies, and that's 100 per cent their choice and should never be judged by anyone. So take the time to make your choices, and ask for help and support if you feel unable to make decisions that are needing to be made.

Fear stalks grief and tries to hijack your feelings. I would go as far as saying it's impossible to encounter loss and not to have to battle with terror on some level, so let me assure you that you are normal if you are fighting with this emotion. You are not mad. You are not losing it. You are on a journey towards healing and, as the darkest layers of grief start to fade and you become more accustomed to living with loss, if you have learnt the skills to battle anxiety, I promise you this: life can move forward with hope.

EXERCISES

Learning to relax is not as easy as it sounds. We live in a world that is full of noise and distractions, and to teach oneself to switch off can be extremely challenging. But I promise you that relaxing the brain and body is something that everyone can learn with commitment and practice.

To me, mindfulness and relaxation are the same things; both are about learning to calm the body and focus on one thing. They are about being present and at peace with oneself.

So how do you get started? You start by mastering basic breathing and relaxation exercises. Once you have learnt the basics, you can move on to more complex exercises. You can practise in your own home, in the great outdoors, even in your car – this is the beauty of relaxation, it can go with you wherever you are.

I like to post a reminder to myself to practise and make myself aware. This may be in the form of a physical note posted on my mirror, or a reminder on my phone, or a diary alert. It is incredible how much tension we carry without even being aware of it. Just taking the time to notice when our muscles are tightening up and our breathing is becoming shallower can make a world of difference.

A few keynotes:
- Before starting any new physical exercise, please seek the advice of your doctor or midwife.
- Following any breathing or physical exercise ensure

you sit up carefully. Ensure you do not feel giddy or lightheaded before moving or driving.

When you are scared or anxious, your muscles carry the stress, and they can become tight and even painful and sore. You may notice knots in your back or shoulders, and you may feel physically tired or exhausted. Stress can often manifest in physical symptoms or illness, so you may also experience pain in your jaw, teeth, tension headaches, or digestive issues such as indigestion.

So your first challenge is to teach your muscles how to relax, and to do that you need to learn to recognise what tension feels like in your body.

Relaxation exercise

Warning – if you have any physical injuries or muscle pain do not tense the muscles in that area as you do not want to exacerbate any injury or condition.

1. From a sitting or lying down position, become aware of how your body feels in this moment. Do you feel tension or tightness in your body, or your face? You don't need to do anything yet, just notice any sensations. Clear your mind of any thoughts, just focus on how you feel physically. Is your heart racing? Notice it. Do you feel tension in parts of your body? Be aware of it. Now remind yourself that stress isn't all negative, it can also bring about positive things too. We aren't wanting to engage in a battle with stress, we just want to settle your mind, calm your spirit and relax in this moment.

2. Close your eyes and take four long deep breaths.

3. Now clench your toes and feet as hard as you can and take a deep breath in.
   - Hold for three to five seconds.

- Then release the breath as you relax the toes and feet.
- Notice the change in feeling and pay attention to how your relaxed muscles feel.

4. Next, tense the muscles in your legs and thighs as hard as you can, while taking a deep breath in.
   - Hold for three to five seconds.
   - As you release the tension, breathe out.
   - Be aware of how different all your muscles feel when they are consciously relaxed.

5. Next, tense the muscles in your fingers and hands, by curling the fingers into tight fists. Squeeze as hard as you can while breathing in.
   - Hold for three to five seconds and release.
   - Then tense all the muscles of your arms on an inhale, and release them on an exhale.
   - Can you feel the tension leaving your body?

6. Next, tense the muscles in your shoulders and neck, while breathing in.
   - Hold for three to five seconds and release on an exhale.

7. Then, tense the muscles in your face. Screw up your eyes, tense your lips.
   - Hold for three to five seconds and release on an exhale.

8. Now, while you are sitting or lying down, focus on the sensation of every muscle being relaxed. Lie/sit here for as long as possible, enjoying the relaxation. Some people have mastered the art of thinking of nothing as they sit in peace; I haven't, so instead I choose to think of a happy memory while staying still for as long as I can. Once I become restless, I stop the exercise and move on with another task or the rest of my day. If you have more time available, try this exercise one limb at a time, so right foot first, then left, and so on.

Grounding techniques

When you are scared or having a panic attack it can be helpful to do grounding exercises. These are techniques that help you to stay in the moment and help you to re-engage with the present. Some grounding exercises are extremely brief, others are longer. Sometimes you may need to do a few different exercises before you feel calmer and back in control.

1. Take 20 deep breaths. Imagine you are slowly blowing up a balloon. Count each breath as you take it. Ensure you inhale deeply, as well as exhaling deeply.
2. Look around you, name 10 things you can see. Smell the air, what can you smell? Reach out, describe what you can feel. Describe what your feet are touching. The challenge here is to focus on your surroundings, which will distract you from panic, and make you feel and be present.
3. Wash your face and focus on the temperature of the water. Watch how the water drips off your hands and washes down the sink. As you dry your hands and face focus on how the towel feels on your skin.
4. Have a drink. Focus on the temperature of the beverage, is it cold or hot? Then focus on the flavour, how would you describe it? Be aware of how it feels as it glides down your throat, and imagine it making its way through your body.
5. If you are with someone, focus on their appearance. How would you describe them? Look at their face, and describe their eyes, their nose, their mouth, their hair. Listen to their voice and focus on their words.
6. Focus on one object or scene in front of you. Describe it in great detail.
7. Describe who you are and what your interests are.
8. Listen – What can you hear? Start with the sounds far away, and then name the things you can hear close by.
9. Put your hands to your face and smell them. What can you smell? Describe the scent.

10. Hold an object in your hands. Focus on how it feels, and
    describe it in your mind.

You can create your own grounding exercises; you don't need
to only use the ones listed.

Breathing exercise

I know teaching you how to breathe sounds silly, as on average
we all breathe in and out between 17,000 and 30,000 times a
day, but it is amazing how shallowly we breathe most of the
time. Recent studies have shown that deep belly breathing
stimulates the vagus nerve, a bundle of nerves that runs from
the head down the neck, through the chest and to the colon.
Stimulating the vagus nerve activates our relaxation response,
slows our heart rate and blood pressure and has been shown
to lower stress levels. So it's worth a try.

Start by sitting or lying down in a comfortable position.
(I prefer to lie down as I find it easier to relax.) I find this
exercise is hard to do when feeling either too hot or too cold.
So if you're hot perhaps use an electric fan, and if you are
cold, wrap yourself in a warm blanket.

- Ensure you have space and quiet, with no distractions
  (I know this can be a challenge in itself!).
- Ensure you feel comfortable.
- Place your left hand on your chest and your right hand
  on your stomach.
- Breathe deeply in through your nose for four seconds.
  Breathe deep down into your abdomen, so that you feel
  your right hand begin to rise with the breath. The left
  hand on your chest should move slightly.
- Hold your breath for five to seven seconds.
- Exhale through your mouth, releasing as much air as you

can, while tightening your abdominal muscles, as if you are squeezing out all the air, for six to eight seconds. Your right hand will fall as you exhale and the abdomen drops, but your other hand will only move slightly.
- Continue to breathe deeply in through your nose and exhale through your mouth.
- Breathe in for four seconds.
- Hold for five to seven seconds.
- Exhale for six to eight seconds.

Once you have mastered the art of deep breathing, you won't need to put your hands on your chest or stomach, as you will be super-aware if you are doing it correctly.

Visualisation exercise

Sit quietly somewhere, pick a place where you are unlikely to be disturbed. In your mind imagine a location. Maybe it's somewhere you have visited in the past, or perhaps it is somewhere you have always dreamt of escaping to. Ensure the location you are thinking of is a place of peace, tranquillity and calm (rather than a bustling city).

Now imagine you are walking around your dream location. Take in every tree, lake, cloud, sea, bird. Focus in on the detail of everything.

- Can you imagine the scent? Breathe it in.
- Can you imagine what the ground feels like beneath your feet? Is it soft or hard? Warm or cold?
- Can you feel the sun on your skin or the chill of the snow?
- Find a place to sit or lie down in your imagined place and practise your breathing exercises. Stay there for 10 to 20 minutes.
- Practise this often, so that you can easily imagine yourself in your safe location when times are stressful.

In nature exercise

Before you practise this exercise, ensure wherever you go is safe, so that you can fully relax.

- Go to a park, garden, woodland or any green space surrounded by nature.
- Turn your phone to silent, so you won't be disturbed.
- Start by doing a couple of minutes of deep breathing.
- Then start to stroll. Don't consider where you are heading; the whole point is to stay in the present.
- Be aware of the trees around you.
- The birds above you.
- The shades of colour surrounding you.
- What can you hear?
- Notice the scent of the air.
- The temperature of the air touching your skin.
- Feel the weight of your body in your feet as they walk across the ground.
- Be aware of any tension in your body.
- Relax your arms, un-tense your fingers.
- Breathe deeply and exhale slowly.
- Enjoy being present in nature.

Self-massage

Giving yourself a hand or foot massage really can bring a sense of calm. I also love doing facial massage on myself as I carry a lot of tension in my jaw. There are some super-useful facial massage videos on YouTube, and by doing these a few times a week, I notice a real difference in the tension I carry in my jaw and neck.

Of course you can also ask your partner or a friend to massage you too, or pay for a professional massage. Just ensure any treatments are safe in pregnancy.

Colouring or craft

Why do people stop colouring as soon as they become adults? And why is this activity considered a creative outlet for children but not for adults? It mystifies me, as it is such a helpful way for people to relax. Colouring can give you a window of time where you think of nothing other than staying within the lines, and which colour to use next. If you loved colouring as a child, let me encourage you to purchase an adult colouring book and a beautiful set of pens, and see if you still love it as an adult. If you adore stationery like me, this is the perfect excuse to head to your nearest store and spoil yourself.

If colouring isn't your thing, there are so many crafts available to us all. I strongly believe that even those who don't consider themselves artistic can find an art form they enjoy and that will relax them – so keep looking until you find your craft of choice.

My top relaxation tips

Find five things to help you relax.

- One to activate your creative talent.
- One to keep you physically fit.
- One to help you rest and sit still.
- One that sparks joy.
- One that inspires you.

Try to practise them all weekly.

YOUR HEALTH IN PREGNANCY

Pregnancy can be beautiful, but it can also be incredibly frustrating, and one can often feel totally out of control, as there seems little you can do to ensure all will end well. But there is plenty of good advice out there, which can help you to feel that you are giving this pregnancy the best possible chance. In this section I'm breaking down some of the current advice, to help ensure you are on the right path.

Diet

Please know the tips below are just guidelines – I took the approach that as long as I ate healthily most of the time, I was doing fine. The most important thing is that you are kind to yourself at this time, not beating yourself up for not following the textbook.

This information is taken from research undertaken immediately before publication, but as guidelines are subject to change, I recommend that you also speak to your midwife to ensure you have the most up-to-date advice.

A balanced diet is an important part of a healthy lifestyle, but it is even more important when pregnant, as the food you eat helps the baby grow. Eating a varied diet helps you and the baby get a good array of nutrients and vitamins. Mums often find they are hungrier than normal, but the old wives' tale that they are eating for two isn't correct (even though the idea of it may be nice). Starting your day with a healthy balanced breakfast can help with energy levels and nausea; it also means you are less likely to need unhealthy snacks to give you an energy boost.

I am a fan of the advice that you should consider all the food you consume over a week, rather than focusing on individual days or meals, as everyone will have days where it's harder to eat balanced meals. Remember – you don't need to stop eating all of your favourite foods, you are just trying to include as many healthy ingredients, and to make as many wise and informed choices as possible.

- Fruit and vegetables are every pregnant person's friend, as they offer loads of vitamins, as well as much-needed fibre, which can help you avoid constipation and piles. If you can consume at least five portions a day, you are doing well.
- Starchy foods are an important source of energy, as they fill you up without containing too many calories. These include bread, potatoes, rice, cereals, maize, pasta, oats, noodles, millet and yams. If you love chips (like I do), oven chips are lower in fat and salt, so are a healthier option.
- Wholegrains, wholewheat pasta and brown rice are better for us all than starchy white foods. Some of us naturally love these wholegrains, and some of us run in the opposite direction when they are on the plate (I am unfortunately in this latter group!), but the more we can all eat these foods, while pregnant or not, the better our diets will be.
- Each day you ideally need to include protein in your diet. Sources of protein include beans, pulses, fish (try to eat two portions a week), eggs, meat, poultry and nuts. If you eat meat, the current advice is that you should avoid liver and try to only eat lean meat. Also make sure all meat and fish is cooked properly, as your risk of food poisoning goes up when you are pregnant.
- Pregnant people aren't advised to eat shark, swordfish or marlin as these larger fish may contain higher levels of mercury, which can damage a developing baby. You should also avoid having more than two portions of oily fish a week, such as salmon, trout, mackerel and herring, because it can contain pollutants.
- For non-vegans or those without dairy intolerance, dairy

foods such as milk, cheese (no unpasteurised cheese though) and yoghurt are great in pregnancy because they contain calcium and other nutrients that you and your baby need. If you can choose low-fat options, these are even better for you.

Just like in everyday life, it's best to avoid sugary foods where possible, but most of us choose to consume these anyway. I took the stance that nothing hurts when consumed in moderation, but be guided by your midwife.

Try to limit the amount of saturated fat you consume – saturated fat is any fat that remains solid at room temperature, such as lard, butter or coconut oil.

My go-to snack when pregnant was a small baked potato. I found if I could avoid ever feeling really hungry, that (slightly) decreased the feeling of nausea, so having snacks that kept acid at bay became my mission. I used to have baked crisps, dry cereal, dried fruits etc. in snack packs in my bag, just in case I got hungry.

Folic acid and other supplements

The more you can get your vitamins and minerals from the foods you eat the better, but when you are pregnant, it may also be helpful to take additional folic acid and supplements, to make sure you are getting everything that you and the baby need.

Alcohol

The Department of Health recommends that women who think they may become pregnant should not drink alcohol at all. Drinking alcohol at any stage of pregnancy can cause harm to your baby. The more you drink, the greater the risk. If you drank small amounts of alcohol before finding out you were pregnant (in the very early stages of pregnancy), the risk to your baby is very low, but if you are worried, please talk to your doctor.

Medications to prevent loss

There are some medications given to women which are believed to help reduce the chance of loss; these include progesterone and baby aspirin. I am asked all of the time whether I would recommend them. Firstly, the only people who should suggest medication to you are your doctor or midwife, so please speak to them before taking any action. Before a doctor prescribes drugs, they need to investigate whether a person has underlying medical conditions, and also investigate why a previous loss may have taken place. If you want to investigate medication options, ask to see a consultant as soon as possible. Current research suggests these medications may only be effective if they are started early on in pregnancy.

Please note that this is general advice. You are probably already racked with nerves and anxiety, and the last thing I want is for you to carry even more stress because you occasionally eat two chocolate bars, a bag of crisps and a tub of ice-cream in one sitting; just try not to do it every day. If you are worried at all about your diet, please sit down with your midwife or doctor and chat with them; they aren't there to judge, and can offer great advice.

TRAVEL IN PREGNANCY

Travel in pregnancy is something I am asked about all the time. If you are feeling nervous, travelling away from home can make you feel genuinely out of your comfort zone. So what advice can I offer?

Firstly, I would suggest that before you make any travel

plans, you should seek advice from your doctor and midwife. They know your medical history better than anyone and can give you reliable information that will hopefully help you to make the best choice for you and your baby.

Here is some general advice that may be helpful to you (please note that none of this advice should be used as a substitute for speaking to your medical team).

1. Talk with your doctor and midwife *before* you book any travel.
2. Ensure you have travel insurance in place and make sure the insurers know you are pregnant. Don't wait until just before you travel to take out a policy; take it out the moment you book your trip, just in case you need to cancel.
3. Consider the medical services on offer in the area you plan on visiting. If you or your baby did need medical help, would you be happy to receive it from the hospital/ doctors in that location?
4. Most airlines will need a fit to fly certificate if you are over 28 weeks of pregnancy, and most don't allow passengers to fly if they are over 36 weeks' gestation. Be really mindful of these dates, as booking a trip at, say, 27 weeks could be risky, if you get stranded in a location.
5. Consider the activities you plan to undertake while away. Will you need to do a lot of walking? Cycling? Climbing? Do you feel able to do them, and does your doctor agree that they are safe for you?
6. If you are going on a flight, be aware that blood clots are more of a risk while pregnant, so take all necessary precautions. Firstly, avoid long flights. Short flights carry less risk. Secondly, wear compression socks and ensure you do regular foot and ankle exercises while in the air and sitting still. Thirdly, drink lots of water. And finally, try to get out of your seat regularly – walk up and down the aisle and stretch if you can.

7. Wear sunscreen. While pregnant, you need to use a much higher factor sunscreen than you perhaps usually use, as you are more at risk of burning or getting pigmentation marks. I recommend using at least factor 50. You need to apply sunscreen on top of any makeup, not under it, as you want it to offer you the most protection possible.

8. Wear a hat if you are in the sun – the last thing you want is sunstroke while pregnant.

9. Take with you all medications you may need. Trying to explain what you need to a pharmacist can be pretty tricky if you don't speak the language (I know of someone who accidentally used deep heat ointment on her haemorrhoids, rather than haemorrhoid cream, due to a language mix-up!).

10. Ensure you stay well hydrated at all times. Drink bottled water if travelling overseas, and remember ice is often made from local water, so ask for drinks with no ice.

11. Be careful about what you eat. This can be tricky when you are away, but if in doubt pick very safe options; it is much better to be safe than sorry.

12. Avoid totally flat shoes as these can cause bad posture and foot pain. Shoes with a slight heel are better for your back and feet while you are pregnant.

13. Pack your favourite snacks, so you know you have things to eat if it turns out the food does not agree with you.

14. Take a photocopy of your medical notes with you.

15. Keep talking to your partner or travel companions about how you feel. At times trips can seem overwhelming, especially if you feel obliged to act happy and 'holidayish' all the time. Make a promise to yourself that you won't fake feeling anything – it is better to be honest with yourself and those you're holidaying with. They will hopefully understand if you need time out, or time alone.

16. Try to enjoy yourself and truly relax; at times, a change of scenery is good for the heart and soul.

SURVEY

I surveyed 232 women who had navigated pregnancy after loss. You may find their answers reflect your own thoughts and worries.

What did you struggle with most in pregnancy (after loss)?

The top 10 answers given were:
1. Terror of bleeding and fearing using the loo.
2. Panic, about everything, but especially about encountering further loss.
3. Inability to relax while pregnant, and a deep, consuming fear that if they did relax, something would go wrong.
4. People not understanding why they couldn't enjoy their pregnancy.
5. The struggle to come to terms with the disappointment that their last pregnancy didn't end up with a child to raise, while pregnant again with another child.
6. Navigating milestones, especially when bad things happened at those points last time.
7. Coping with the panic every time they felt any ache or pain.
8. The horror of having to constantly explain about their previous loss(es) to new medical people.
9. Never getting to enjoy the pregnancy or planning, as in the back of their mind they didn't believe they would bring their baby home.
10. The dread of scans, in case they are told bad news, but at the same time, the scans could bring temporary reassurance that their baby was OK.

I think anyone navigating pregnancy after a loss will relate to most, if not all, of the things in this list. The irony is, when you are feeling like this, you feel so alone, and are worried you are the only person dealing with it. I hope that seeing this list in black and white will show you that any fears and worries you are encountering are 100 per cent normal. I asked these ladies:

Was your doctor helpful in offering support to you in pregnancy post-loss?

Yes 35.78% No 64.22%
Sadly, I am not surprised that 64 per cent of people felt that their doctor failed to give them support in pregnancy, as I hear this regularly from individuals. I hope in the future this will change as training gets better, and loss becomes more understood.

Was your midwife helpful in offering support to you in pregnancy post-loss?

Yes 43.97% No 56.03%
This is an unfortunate result and, again, I can only hope that time and training will change this.

Did another grief wave hit you post-delivery?

Yes 62.07% No 37.93%
I hear from so many people each week who wish they had been warned that they might experience a new wave of grief once their baby is born. When you have a baby in your arms, you hope the only feeling you will be hosting is an abundance of joy but, for many people, another grief wave hits them shortly after delivery. It happens for many reasons.

1. Having a baby in your arms can make you think of the babies who should be here with you but aren't.
2. Your hormones go haywire following giving birth, and emotions are high.

3. Women are often exhausted following having a baby, and when they are tired, grief can become more apparent.
4. Mothers often worry that the world will see their new baby as a replacement for the one that has died, and that causes such panic that it brings a new layer of grief to the surface.
5. Being around hospitals, midwives, doctors etc. can be a trigger that reminds a person of past experiences.
6. If a person is suffering with post-traumatic stress, giving birth can be a trigger, and can bring with it grief and other feelings.
7. Some people don't allow themselves to fully grieve until they have another baby in their arms – they almost put their grief on pause. Once their next baby has arrived safely, it can feel like a weight has been lifted, and their grief journey begins for the baby they previously lost.

There are many other reasons, of course, but these seem to be the most common.

Were you able to feel joy in pregnancy?

Yes 49.57%   No 50.43%
Sadly, so many people lose the ability to feel joy in pregnancy after loss. This happens mostly due to the anxiety a person is battling daily. I hope that this book helps anyone who is struggling to discover the joy in their pregnancy.

Did the fear you encountered in pregnancy then transfer to fearing for your baby's life once they were born?

Yes 67.67%   No 32.33%
We don't talk about this enough. It certainly took me by surprise when Esmé arrived in my arms. I presumed the worry would end once my child was safely delivered; I wasn't

prepared for the anxiety to continue in a different guise. This is why it is imperative to challenge the fear in pregnancy and develop skills and tricks to overcome it.

Do you still battle with anxiety about your child's health or well-being?

Yes 66.38%   No 33.62%
While I accept it's 100 per cent normal to be anxious about one's children, I think most parents who have encountered loss will worry that little bit more. There are ways to control this anxiety and fear, and I would encourage anyone and everyone to try to manage the panic and stress, as life is far less enjoyable if you are walking around with an umbrella, just in case it rains!

Did the fear of loss dictate how many children you decided to have?

Yes 52.16%   No 47.84%
I am surprised this is pretty much an even split, I would have expected it to be more like 70 per cent yes. It just goes to show that when it comes to love, people are genuinely willing to risk their hearts and emotions, and I am so glad they are.

Did friends and family understand the fear you carried in pregnancy?

Yes 35.62%   No 64.38%
This result doesn't surprise me. I think fear and loss are pretty hard to understand and grasp unless you have walked through that valley yourself.

I hope these results show you that you are not alone in how you may be feeling.

PREGNANCY ADVENT

Here is a picture to colour in, it is my version of a Christmas advent calendar. Each week you get to colour in a number. There are 40 numbers, as an average pregnancy is 40 weeks in length. As the picture becomes more colourful, it's a visual example of how far you have travelled.

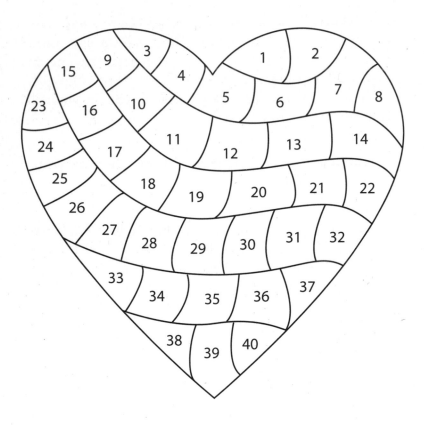

PART 2

Support and Journalling

Weekly Support

The weekly support offered on these pages begins at week five of gestation. I am aware that some of you will have purchased this book before you are even expecting, so it may be sitting on your bedside table on the day you discover you are pregnant. For you, this book will journey with you from the moment you see a positive on a pregnancy test stick (often discovered at the end of four weeks' gestation). Others will purchase this book further on in pregnancy, so I have chosen not to lay it out in pre-set gestation sections. Instead I have put together 36 weeks of support, starting from gestational week five, through to week 40. If you are starting the book when you are eight weeks pregnant, I would advise you to read the first four weeks in one or two sittings, and then move forward to join the daily practice at the right point.

When I started writing this book, I had planned to do a straightforward week-by-week guide to pregnancy rather than a daily guide. Following a long chat with my friend Rachel who had suffered from prenatal depression due to severe hyperemesis, I decided I needed to do daily support, as each day feels so long when you are pregnant. I know I needed a friend to walk alongside me; my hope is this book will become your companion, and that knowing you have a reason to dip into the pages each morning or evening will help you get through the next nine months.

I considered adding in a separate section for partners, but after discussing what to include in it with Andy, I quickly discovered his fears had been exactly the same as mine.

He was terrified every time I had gone to the loo. He had lain awake at night fretting that scans were approaching. So I felt that to include a small section for partners was almost insulting, as though it implied they may feel less or differently than the person carrying the baby, and for the majority of people pregnancy is something you experience together as a couple. So every section in this book is for both parents. Of course some parts may not apply to one party, but I hope by reading it all, it will help bring further understanding and offer support to anyone who needs it.

There is something I have to address, even though I would rather not, and that is what happens if you lose your precious baby while working through this book. I would suggest you then keep this book and journal as a beautiful reminder of your baby, along with scan photos (if you have them) or other mementos you have saved. I would love to have had something like this to look back on with the children I lost; it would be a very special keepsake. If a loss happens, I recommend reading my earlier book, *The Baby Loss Guide*. This will offer vital information and support to help navigate through the pain and grief. Now I have addressed that, let us move on.

You will see that each of the seven days is carefully structured around a weekly plan that combines support, advice and exercises. I urge you to complete the tasks, especially the journalling exercises, as you will only receive the benefit by physically doing the tasks.

I have included journalling as it is a great way to process stress and worry. Some say it is as powerful a tool as face-to-face talking and therapy, which is fantastic as it doesn't depend on a third party. Here are the ways journalling has been shown to help people when it is done regularly.

Journalling helps you to:

- manage anxiety
- reduce stress levels and practise relaxation

- cope with depression and mental health conditions
- improve and stabilise a positive mindset
- process concerns
- navigate issues, and identify fear, panic and trauma triggers
- identify symptoms that are being experienced and find patterns of feelings
- improve focus on positive outcomes and solutions
- allow pain and feelings to be heard, expressed and processed

I hope, whether this is the first time you have tried journalling or whether you are well-practised at it, the exercises will be something you enjoy and find to be therapeutic and beneficial.

GRATITUDE JOURNALLING

Each day concludes with space to write in something you are grateful for.

Today I am grateful for

Why is this important?

Neuroscientists have found that being thankful and showing gratitude can literally help you to be happier. The simple act of focusing on what is good in your life can make you feel more optimistic about the future. But it doesn't stop there: those who practise gratitude journalling have even been shown to benefit physically. People report better sleep quality, less fatigue, reduced levels of anxiety and depression, and many other benefits. It is truly amazing to see both the short-term and long-term effects of practising something so simple.

I have personally seen the benefits of gratitude in my own life. I truly believe this practice (which took me a little time to cultivate) transformed my life. It helped me come to terms with my losses and helped me process my grief, and it then helped me navigate pregnancy after loss. It is amazing how the focus of your day changes when you start looking out for things to be grateful for. Eventually your brain almost gets rewired and you start looking for the positives rather than the negatives in every situation. I hope over the coming weeks you enjoy this task and may perhaps keep doing it once you have completed this book.

The week at a glance

Day one is always a support day, offering insight or a thought about a topic.

Day two is a practical task.

Day three is either a personal story from someone who has experienced a pregnancy post-loss, or an expert sharing their knowledge. For some these personal stories of loss and pregnancy will make them feel less alone and will offer them reassurance, while for others they could be a panic trigger. Only you know you, so if they help you, please read them; if they don't help you simply skip them each week and perhaps read them when your baby is safely in your arms. All of the personal stories are in a grey box, so they are easy to spot, and easy to avoid if that's what you choose to do.

Day four is another support day, offering insight or a thought about a topic.

Day five is for journalling about your pregnancy and also offers a quote that I hope will resonate with you.

Day six is another support day, offering insight or a thought about a topic.

Day seven is a journalling day, where I ask you questions which I hope will make you think and reflect. The week concludes with another quote that I hope touches your soul.

So let's get started!

WEEK 5

DAY 1

Support – Grief triggers

Occasions that trigger your grief can often blindside you. They are hard enough to handle in ordinary life, let alone when pregnant. Let me reassure you that just because something is a grief trigger now, doesn't mean it will always be one. Down the line, your trigger may become a beautiful reminder, rather than a powerful blow to the stomach.

So what are some common grief triggers?

- Occasions – Christmas, holidays, Mother's and Father's Day, etc.
- Certain dates – death anniversaries, funeral dates, due dates, birthdays, etc.
- Music
- Food
- Places – hospitals, doctors' surgeries, shops, restaurants, hotels, and specific locations
- Baby bumps, pregnancy announcements or seeing babies
- Times of day or days of the week
- Using the bathroom

How does one cope with triggers?

If something you do every day is a trigger, especially things you do repeatedly each day (such as using the bathroom), you may want to seek professional help to disable/disarm it, so you don't feel you are being held captive by it.

Avoidance of a trigger is often assumed to be the easiest way of avoiding being deeply affected. While avoidance can at times be useful and healthy, at other times it's not an option. If your life is being restricted and the world you reside in is getting smaller (for example, if there is a list of places you now struggle to visit), you may want to deal with the trigger, and remove its power to bring you to your knees.

How do you face a trigger head-on? If you feel able to face your triggers, or if you are unable to avoid them (such as seeing a midwife, for example), try to plan how you will deal with it. Perhaps you need to prepare a set answer if someone asks you something. Maybe you need to plan your reply if tears do start to fall, so you don't feel any embarrassment. Perhaps you need to have an exit plan if the occasion gets too much for you to handle – things like this can help you navigate emotionally challenging situations.

Pick your battles and focus on the biggest triggers first. Some may be easy to avoid and have no consequence on life if you miss them (such as going to a friend's dinner party), while other things do affect us or those around us if we extract ourselves from them (such as attending your niece's christening), so it's worth spending time freeing yourself from those triggers first.

What can you do if you are overwhelmed by grief?

- Try to take a few moments to be alone (if possible).
- Take some deep breaths, and reassure yourself that you will survive this moment, that these feelings will pass. Speak to yourself as you would speak to a friend or a child – with love and compassion, not judgement. Use the techniques in the exercise section.
- Have a playlist on your phone with soothing music, or a mindfulness app that allows you to escape into your head for a while, or visit https://www.thewaitingroom.life/
- If the place and time allow, permit yourself to let the tears flow. Sometimes all you need is a good cry, and that allows the feelings you are experiencing to be less overwhelming.

- If you choose to avoid processing the emotions until a later date, I want to encourage you to revisit the feelings. Grief, pain and trauma will always resurface. If you can deal with the emotions in moments chosen by you – perhaps in your home chatting with a partner or friend, or maybe in a room with a counsellor – it's a lot easier than being forced to deal with it at a traumatic or public moment.

Today I am grateful for

DAY 2

Task

Write a note to your baby – What do you want to tell them about you? What are your interests, what are your hopes and dreams for you (not them)?

Today I am grateful for

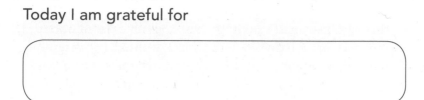

DAY 3

Sarah's Story

After we lost our first baby, all I wanted was to be pregnant again. I couldn't bear the empty feeling. Having experienced the miscarriage while travelling in Africa, we were given some wildly contradictory advice on when we should – or could – start trying again. The doctors in Zimbabwe told me it wasn't safe to get pregnant again within the next six months. My heart sank. Six months felt forever. Online forums said three months, or one month, or whatever feels right for you. It was confusing, especially in my vulnerable emotional state.

I was scared of losing another baby. I was scared of somehow damaging my womb and negatively affecting my fertility.

Then there was the mother in me; I didn't want to betray the sweet little life that we'd lost. The life that wasn't mine to hold, to watch grow. I wanted to honour their memory, and I didn't want to feel like we were rushing to 'replace' them. But I also didn't want to mourn in a way that meant not trying for another sweet little life. I was ready for our family to grow.

My husband and I, out on our travels, talked for hours and hours, every day. Luckily, we were on the same page about everything, and that's partly what helped me get through. I wanted to talk in every possible detail about our first little baby – so did he. I wanted to imagine what they might have done, cry about the injustice of what they'd never do – so did he. I wanted to keep hope alive, talking about the children we would hold in our arms – so did he. The talking helped. It helped so much. And, in talking, we decided there was no reason to wait some randomly prescribed amount of time. We would always love our first baby – our Little Adventurer as we named them, since they'd joined us in four countries on our travels. We'd always love them for making us parents, for showing us how fiercely we could love someone we'd never met. It didn't matter if their sibling came soon after or we waited a year. It didn't change the love we felt for our first child.

So, once my cycle stabilised and my body no longer registered as 'pregnant' on tests (I found that part so bitterly cruel), we saw no reason to wait. And, to my complete surprise and delight, I was pregnant that first month of trying again.

I felt elated but, obviously, in a different way to my first pregnancy. The naïvety was gone. The pure optimism was gone. I felt fragile. The child inside me felt like the most fragile thing in the world.

At eight weeks pregnant I had a small bleed and my heart fell through my body and my lungs filled with lead. I knew, in my rational mind, that bleeding can be completely normal, but women who've gone through a miscarriage know that you watch for any sign that your happiness might be ripped away. Your happiness has no tangibility to it. Especially in those first 12 weeks before a scan. You're falling more and more in love with a tiny, growing person who you're overjoyed to meet one day but terrified in case you never do.

Wanting to know as soon as possible whether everything was OK with our baby, I phoned a doctor and she was very kind and reassuring, booking me in for an emergency scan at the earliest opportunity: the next morning. I remember a fitful night, unable to relax without knowing if the baby inside me, the baby I already loved so dearly, was alive or not.

My husband, Jonny, clutched my hand as the sonographer looked for a heartbeat. It seemed to take her an age. And her face, emotionless, gave nothing away. Even as a lifelong optimist, I feared the worst. The longer she took, looking for a heartbeat, the more this felt like the heartbreak of our scan in Zimbabwe.

So we waited for her to speak. To say anything.

'There are two sacs but I'm not seeing a heartbeat yet,' the sonographer said.

'Oh no, there's one.'

'. . . And there's the other.'

At first, I didn't understand. We'd gone in thinking it was a binary outcome: was our baby alive or not? Instead we'd come face to face with a third outcome that had never crossed my mind: twins.

I was overjoyed. I felt like we had won the lottery, without even buying a ticket. I forgot twins were even a thing that could happen if you were pregnant. I looked at Jonny as he squeezed my hand and we both cried happy, ecstatic tears.

For some, I can imagine finding out you're having twins might feel overwhelming, not what you wanted, a scary prospect. I felt nothing but excitement and pure, pure joy. Yes, there were now two tiny lives to worry about, but it felt right. We were going to be twin parents. I felt born for the role.

One of the best things about a twin pregnancy is you

have far more regular scans, one every month. Those helped me no end. I never had to go more than four weeks without seeing my babies and, experiencing this pregnancy after loss, I was so incredibly grateful for each scan. Each reassuring glimpse of my wriggling bubbas.

Jonny found the scans harder than I did. Like I said, I'm an eternal optimist. Although I'm capable of imagining the worst, something in me always clings to the best-case scenario. As the man, not carrying the babies and not able to control the fate of his wife or children, Jonny found the scans stressful. The Zimbabwean one always played on his mind. Each time he'd prepare himself to hear that one twin, or both, hadn't made it. But that wasn't the case. And, as time went on and they got bigger and stronger, with fully formed organs and features, we found ourselves relaxing more and more. These were the children we would meet, hold, teach, love in person.

I didn't feel either baby kick until I was over five months pregnant. The doctors explained that I might not, as I had an anterior placenta (at the front) which cushioned any movements until they were bigger. I remember where I was when I felt that incredible first kick: sat in my favourite bookshop, reading a baby name book. A friend asked me afterwards, 'Well, which name did they kick for?', but I'd been too thrilled to notice. I can't explain how real those kicks made my babies feel to me. It was one of the best moments of my life. From then on, like so many expectant couples, our favourite way to spend an evening was slouched in front of the TV, ignoring whatever was on and excitedly waiting for the next tiny knee or tiny elbow to make an appearance. With four tiny knees and four tiny elbows to poke my tummy out, we never had too long to wait.

Our twins arrived safely; we got our family. And we still talk about our Little Adventurer. We can't wait to visit the thriving fig tree we planted in Zimbabwe where their tiny body is buried.

It's the strangest feeling to know that, if our first baby had lived, we'd never have had our hilarious, wonderful and darling twins, conceived during those nine months.

We will tell our twins that their hugely loved, always-remembered older sibling stepped aside so that they could be born.

Today I am grateful for

DAY 4

Support – When you feel only fear rather than joy

You spend months or possibly years trying to get pregnant, and when you finally see those pink lines on the pregnancy test, you feel very little joy; you just feel terror! How can that be? This is the moment you have been waiting for, begging for, longing for! You are then not only feeling panic; you are also feeling a shedload of guilt.

This is not how it played out in your imagination. You were meant to be jumping up and down with excitement. You were supposed to be planning how to reveal this amazing news to your partner. But no, here you are, shaking in the bathroom and wanting to vomit because you feel so terrified.

Let me tell you all of this is normal!

It is perfectly possible to have wanted something for your whole life, and still fall apart when you get it.

When your brain is overwhelmed, and it can't even comprehend how it will navigate the anxiety for the next eight and a half months, it is natural to panic. So please don't feel any guilt if you had this reaction. It does not mean you will be a bad mother; you will be an amazing mother. It does not mean your baby felt any rejection; they will only feel love.

Your new reality just takes time to process, so give yourself time to come to terms with this wonderful, life-changing news.

I will conclude this with a quote from my daughter Esmé, as I feel it is so apt and spot-on.

· ·

When you start to feel frightened,
all the good things vanish from your head.

· · · · · · · · · · · ESMÉ CLARK-COATES (AGE 10) · · · · · · · · · · ·

We need to try to hold on to the good things and remind ourselves to feel the joy, even when fear makes them so hard to see.

For some the fear of repeated loss is so consuming that the only way they can handle pregnancy after loss is to almost go into denial that it is happening. They refuse to acknowledge it or talk about it. If this is your way of surviving the early months of pregnancy that is totally OK. As long as you are following all healthcare advice, and attend the medical appointments that are necessary for your health and the baby's, that is fine. My belief is whatever helps you make it through is good. No one should feel guilty for doing it their way; this is your journey, you design the path you take.

Today I am grateful for

DAY 5

Journalling your pregnancy

What gestation is your baby today? _____

How big are they? _____

What symptoms are you now feeling?

What do you want to remember about how you are feeling or what you are experiencing?

There are seasons when we break,
and times when we heal.
There are valleys that destroy us,
and mountains that build us.
The secret to surviving?
Simple! Know that there is no secret . . .
There is no fast pass and no hidden tunnel
to escape the pain.
You just have to face it, breathe it, weep through it,
and then one day you look up and realise the sun has risen
when you thought it would be dark forever.

ZOË CLARK-COATES

Today I am grateful for

DAY 6

Support – Why do we say our heart hurts?

Often those who are grieving say their heart aches, but why is this when feelings don't come from the heart, they are formed and created by the brain? Why don't we all say our minds are full of pain? Or our brain is breaking rather than our heart?

I guess it is because we have all accepted that our hearts are where love is stored and carried. So when a loss happens, we see it as our heart breaking rather than our brains. Research has shown, however, that our minds and hearts are indeed connected, and emotions such as grief and fear can cause substantial heart damage. So how is the damage caused? Dr Sandeep Jauhar, a well-respected heart consultant, explains: 'The nerves that control unconscious processes, such as the heartbeat, can sense the distress and trigger a maladaptive fight-or-flight response that triggers blood vessels to constrict, the heart to gallop and blood pressure to rise, resulting in damage.' This shows us grief can be a heart issue – but it doesn't address why the brain is continuously ignored by us as humans.

By purely focusing on the heart and not addressing the damaging effect fear and grief have on the brain, I believe we are failing mankind. We are making grief seem like an innocent and somewhat weak emotion that can be overcome with a little effort, rather than seeing it as an incredibly powerful force that has the capability to destroy and change lives. It can cause significant trauma, change personalities and hold people captive for years, if not decades.

I believe we need not only to look at the losses people have encountered and help them process the grief associated with them, but also to address the psychological fallout from facing an emotional brain trauma. We need to help people turn their worlds the right way around and help them navigate life on the other side of loss.

You can never fill the hole that someone's passing has created, but you aren't meant to fill it. That space was theirs and theirs alone. What you can do is cover that hole, that cavern, with love and kindness, so they create a seal over it. As new people arrive in your life, your heart will then just expand so they too can be loved by you.

Today I am grateful for

DAY 7

Journal

What are some of your grief triggers? And how do you plan to handle them when they arise?

It's a gift to the soul
if another person
wants to discover
the stitches that hold
together a person's heart.

ZOË CLARK-COATES

Today I am grateful for

WEEK 6

DAY 1

Support – Is it normal to do a lot of pregnancy tests?

I am currently trying to do maths in my head to count how many tests I did; let's just say a lot. It is 100 per cent normal to do a lot of tests and to doubt every one of them. I would say at some point you probably do need to accept that those two pink lines are visible, and you are in fact pregnant, as you don't want to go broke purchasing tests!

When you want something so badly, it's hard to believe your eyes when the test confirms you are pregnant. I used to have a sterile jar by the loo to collect my first morning urine in, so I could keep re-testing with the same sample. Yes, I was indeed a pregnancy test pro!

Those minutes when you are sitting and waiting, and your heart is racing, are hard to describe. You want to look, but you are too scared to watch. Then when you finally check, and it's a faint positive . . . You shake. You cry. You decide you need to re-test.

So why do some tests show a fainter positive than others? I am assuming this is due to the amount of dye in the test stick, and also down to how sensitive the stick is. But a positive is a positive, and you should ignore how dark the line is showing. If you are getting an inconclusive result, change brands, as some are well known for being less sensitive than others, or ask your doctor to test for you.

People always ask me if they are weird to continue doing pregnancy tests daily. I reassure them they are not strange; they are just terrified.

So why do people keep doing repeated pregnancy tests?

They simply can't believe what they are seeing. But they also want to ensure they are still pregnant. Anxiety torments us with thoughts like, *Just because you were pregnant yesterday, doesn't mean you are today.* After loss it is super-common to lose faith in one's body; most people fear they don't have the ability to create and hold on to their offspring, and whenever they see those lines on the pregnancy test, it is a visual reminder that right now things are still OK, so they get a few moments of relief from the fear.

At some point, however, you do need to stop testing, as it not only costs you a fortune, but also encourages the terror to take hold. Every day you are putting yourself through a big-dipper ride of uncertainty and fear, while you wait for the test to confirm positive. This encourages the fight-or-flight response to stay on high alert, which in turn makes you constantly on the edge of panic. Try to stop testing and start accepting. You are pregnant, and let me be one of the first to congratulate you.

Today I am grateful for

DAY 2

Task

Spend time thinking of what you are most proud of yourself for and create a list. I appreciate for some this is a tough challenge. It's often easier to criticise oneself than to sit back and acknowledge one's achievements, but have a go.

Today I am grateful for

DAY 3

Dr Jacque Gerrard MBE, Midwife Consultant and former Director for England at the Royal College of Midwives

How would you suggest someone navigate worry when pregnant again following a loss?

It is important that maternity services provide parent-led, sensitive and empathic care for all parents, but particularly those who have suffered baby loss. Midwives are skilled listeners and advocates for women and will be aware that anxieties are heightened following baby loss, particularly in a subsequent pregnancy. Women must always be encouraged to talk to their midwife, let them know their worries, anxieties and concerns. If the model of care is one of continuity, then the midwife will be tuned in to a woman's emotions.

Why do some people get pregnancy symptoms, such as morning sickness, and others don't?

Around 80 per cent of women get morning sickness. All women are individuals, and all pregnancies are different, so some get pregnancy symptoms, and others don't. Some women get severe morning sickness, while others get none. In the vast majority of cases, the sickness subsides at around 16 weeks.

Today I am grateful for

DAY 4

Support – Why and how?

'How can one survive and flourish with so many uncertainties?' This is a question I get asked hundreds of times a week by pregnant ladies. Most are still confused as to why they previously encountered loss, and they are unsure about how they will survive the next eight months of pregnancy, with so much anxiety to contend with. I wish I could tell you there was a magic secret, that all you need to do is XYZ and the worry will vanish, but, of course, I can't tell you this – there isn't any secret.

All you can do is live each day as it comes and try not to look too far ahead.

I can almost hear you saying, 'That's easier said than done, Zoë,' and I agree! It's super-difficult, and there may be days where you have no clue how you will manage, but I promise you will. You will cope, and you will survive. No one feels they can deal with it; I didn't think I could, but I did and so will you.

Today I am grateful for

DAY 5

Journalling your pregnancy

What gestation is your baby today? _____

How big are they? _____

What symptoms are you now feeling?

What do you want to remember about how you are feeling or what you are experiencing?

We aren't supposed to know what to do.
We are meant to feel our way in the darkness.
As we explore, we discover that beauty lies
in the hidden locations, in the unexpected
rooms, in the places we would have never
entered if we hadn't been lost in the first place.

ZOË CLARK-COATES

Today I am grateful for

DAY 6

Support – When worry and fear dominate

If fear was a character in a book, this is what I imagine it
would look like . . .

*Fear – looks like a shadow; it carries a weapon which
throws lines with hooks on, and they can hit everything
in sight. It can disguise itself as a million different things,
like a chameleon, so often you aren't even aware fear
and worry are present. Fear is scared of everything; it is
even scared of itself. Fear is the master of 'what if' . . . It
robs you of peace, as even if things seem OK right now,
it hurtles a 'what if this x happens?' at you, which can
blindside you. It makes you scared of life when things
are both bad and good, as it whispers, 'It won't stay
good for long, so you'd better prepare yourself for pain.'*

Past trauma and life circumstance can change the shape and scale of fear – for some, fear is a small creature that can be quickly demolished. For others, fear is enormous; it's grown throughout their lives, and it is now this massive force that seems to control everything. Often those who have known childhood trauma have the most prominent fears. If they learnt that the monster under the bed is real and not just fictitious, fear can become a colossal part of their story as they journey through life. Additionally, those who learnt to carry fear as a child are more likely to accept it's now part of their everyday lives, as they have journeyed with it since childhood. It's almost become part of who they are, and they can't imagine life without being afraid.

Fear often comes in through the door where grief enters. There is a reason people say that grief is like fear, and that's because where grief resides fear also sits. When you lose someone, you are naturally mourning their departure, but you also fear that you will never feel that love or connection again.

- You may fear feeling lost and in crippling pain forever.
- You may fear never feeling joy again.
- You may fear feeling out of control.
- You may fear encountering more loss in the future (as who would ever want to go through that hell again!).
- You may fear for your health or that of those around you. Your brain could be telling you that if the bottom has fallen from your world once, surely that means it could happen again.
- You may fear going to sleep, as you know when you wake, your reality won't have changed, and it can feel like encountering the loss all over again each morning.

There are so many more things I could write here, but you get the gist. Fear and worry can be crippling and controlling. So how can you stop them from suffocating you?

Different solutions will work for different people, but talking offers the key to freedom for many. As well as therapy and sharing from the heart, there are practical steps people can attempt to do to disarm the power of fear and worry in one's life. For some it will work, for others it won't, but you will only know by trying.

The first step I advise taking is this:

Most people hate feeling worried and afraid, and when those feelings dominate their emotions, they feel anxious and annoyed that they can't stop their minds from going to those dark places. But did you know that the more you try to prevent your brain from worrying, the more it worries? Our brains don't respond well to being told not to think something; in fact, the brain does the exact opposite. The more you try not to feel anxious, the more you fret. So give yourself full permission to think whatever; nothing is off the table. The moment you stop fighting your thoughts, the brain stops freaking out. For example, the thought pops into your head, 'What if something is wrong with this baby?' Try not to dissect this thought, or overanalyse it. Simply acknowledge it. Think to yourself, 'OK, that's what my brain is currently worried about. I can't reassure it right now, but I hope and trust that this baby is fine.' Focus on breathing, and keeping calm when the concerns show their ugly heads, and eventually the panic and fear should settle.

Today I am grateful for

DAY 7

Journal

My worry right now is

I am going to try to overcome this worry by doing

....

People often think those who have been
through trauma and loss are more vulnerable,
but they couldn't be more wrong.
Those who have walked through the fire come
out as warriors and are the best equipped to throw
water on the flames surrounding others.

. . . . ZOË CLARK-COATES . . . .

Today I am grateful for

WEEK 7

• •

DAY 1

Support – Pregnancy symptoms coming and going

Thanks to my overactive imagination, I found I was analysing every possible symptom or lack of symptoms. My doctor was excellent and was able to give me so much reassurance, but I know many are not in that fortunate position. So what do you do if you need that reassurance? You keep asking for it. If your midwife or doctor fails to support you emotionally, it is OK to ask either to move teams or for an additional person who can offer you what you need. I also recommend you try to find a pregnancy buddy who gets what you are feeling. Having another person to share your worries with can help.

Remember, most pregnancy symptoms do come and go; you can have good days and bad days. Tiredness, for instance, had a dramatic impact on my pregnancy sickness, so some days I would feel terribly nauseous, while on others I felt OK. Most days I would feel achy pain, almost like period pains, and my doctor was able to reassure me this was just everything growing and stretching, but it's easy to panic and worry that this is a sign of impending loss.

So my top tip is to talk. Talk to your doctor/midwife. Talk to friends/family/your pregnancy buddy about your worries. Be aware that symptoms do fluctuate and, instead of worrying in silence, go and get checked out, so you can relax.

Today I am grateful for

DAY 2

Task

Write a letter to your baby; what do you want to say to them?

Dear

Today I am grateful for

DAY 3

Lindsay's Story

Persevering with tea-drinking when I was pregnant was more for social purposes than any kind of nutrition or hydration. I was quite literally sick of not being able to stomach anything during meetups with my friends. It seemed the old wives' tales were somewhat warranted: for the fourth time, pregnancy had put me off my favourite cuppa.

Forcing myself to keep drinking tea, all the while hating it, was part of an unwanted and unexpected paradox: the more 'problems' I encountered, the happier I became in myself.

It seemed anything that could find its way into a maternity guide under the heading 'possible challenges faced in pregnancy' was then subsequently filed in my subconscious as 'proof that I must still be pregnant'.

But I wasn't always like this.

During my first pregnancy, the nausea was nothing but a burden interrupting my joy. I was in my final year at university, my first year of marriage, and nothing about spending half of every day in a college bathroom felt reassuring. Not even sharing a diagnosis of hyperemesis with Mariah Carey could persuade me to feel positive about my morning, afternoon and evening sickness. Despite that, and repeated hospital admissions to replace lost fluids, I was so thrilled to be pregnant, and so full of hope and expectation for my unborn child, that I willed myself into maternity clothes. Any twinges, aches and pains, odd feelings or sensations were simply written off as part and parcel of growing a tiny human.

One day, which started with me in a pair of

ridiculously unnecessary mum-to-be trousers, also involved scrambling around for some ginger biscuits (the results of a Google search) to quell my unending nausea. I remember it because it was the morning of our very first scan.

It's a lot more likely that the heavy, nauseating feeling I remember from that day actually set in *after* the scan; after the moment the news was broken to us that our much-longed-for baby had died, likely some weeks earlier.

In an instant, I blamed myself. What had I done? What could have happened? Had I spent so much time enjoying pregnancy that I had forgotten my baby? And the fear that formed the deepest roots: what kind of mother doesn't even know when her own baby has died? At war with myself, I vowed that if I were ever lucky enough to be pregnant again, I would pay more attention to my body, and my baby.

There would be another two pregnancies after this one, both of which would end far too early. By the time number four rolled around any optimism was largely eclipsed by cynicism.

It was such a far cry from when we first sat down as newlyweds imagining our future together. It wasn't so much that we were full of untethered hope and possibility; it was that we had absolutely no frame of reference that would cause us to worry.

Even as a journalist covering health and well-being, I wasn't encumbered by reports on miscarriage. So it never occurred to me as I read pregnancy book after pregnancy book that baby loss would be part of our journey.

One morning at work I was offered a cup of tea; one sip and I found myself driving to Sainsbury's for a pregnancy test. This time a small blue cross emerged, confirming that I was once again pregnant.

Because of my history with loss, I was booked in for an early scan, and at just five weeks pregnant I saw a little flickering peanut on the screen before me. A baby. With a heartbeat. For a split second, I allowed myself to be happy before diving straight back into self-preservation mode.

I became obsessed with counting down days to each new week and spent an inordinate amount of time asking the internet for answers.

At 12 weeks, I had an official scan and dared to ring my mum afterwards to share the news that I'd passed that first major milestone. Letting my guard down ever so slightly, for the first time in that pregnancy, I started looking for nursery furniture. Sitting down with a catalogue and a cup of tea, I quietly sipped as I browsed. Then it dawned on me. An immediate cold sweat broke out, my heart pounded, and I could barely speak. The tea wasn't making me feel sick anymore. Panicking and hyperventilating, I immediately thought the worst. In that moment I was arrested by the possibility that, in being able to tolerate my cup of tea, my body must be telling me I had lost the baby again.

I don't want to skip to the end of the story, but you need to know at this point that pregnancy number four went full term and into the world came my baby boy, Corban.

What I hadn't realised, and couldn't fathom for fear, was that I hadn't reached that point in any of my previous pregnancies. I didn't recognise an uncharted place of wellness and peace.

I had yet to become accustomed to *enjoying* being pregnant.

Sadly, I experienced another very early miscarriage

after Corban, before becoming pregnant once more with my second son, Micah.

That pregnancy, however, looked very different.

I had learnt so much through multiple miscarriages, but perhaps the most poignant lesson was simply to refuse to allow my joy to be stolen. I realised I spent almost my entire pregnancy with Corban living in fear. It's completely ridiculous, but I even asked the doctor seconds after Corban was born if he had a brain! I had allowed every irrational fear to inhabit the spaces once filled with hope, faith, peace and possibility.

On entering my sixth pregnancy, I made a promise to myself that I would enjoy every second of it, however long the pregnancy lasted.

Every pain would be a reminder of the privilege I'd had to mother seven babies altogether (including a lost baby after Micah).

I banned tea and digestives and opted instead for fancy presses, cream cakes and uplifting movies, and I adopted a mantra of 'take every thought captive'.

When I started down the old track of worry and anxiety, I stopped myself and began imagining the days with my babies that lay ahead.

I learnt to love the smallest of movements and flutterings, and treasured the times I had with just me and my bump. I even looked forward to my bi-weekly blood tests dealing with the unwanted and itchy cholestasis. The 20-minute journey and the walk to and from the bus stop allowed me the chance to walk past several reflective shop fronts. With every passing week, I would admire my growing bump.

Whether I was to be mum to Micah for a few short weeks or until I reached 100 years old, I determined to love him and to love my pregnancy.

When I finally realised that motherhood began long before I ever held my children in my arms, it became easier to replace fear with a protective love, and allow pregnancy post-loss to be a daily journey embracing possibility once more.

There's every reason to be hopeful. Every reason to be excited. As the old saying goes, 'love casts out fear'. Learning to love my time as 'mum in waiting' was nothing short of a game-changer.

Today I am grateful for

DAY 4

Support – Friendships

If you are reading this book, it is because you have already gone through the big friendship test . . . baby loss. So you may have already lost and gained some friendships.

I call loss 'the Great Life Sieve' as it really does bring a lot of things to the surface. We learn who is meant to be in our lives through better and worse, and who isn't. Some people simply can't handle loss and grief, and they run away from it, which can make those who are encountering it feel utterly abandoned.

If you have been through this, firstly let me say how sorry I am. It is so hard to lose your friends on top of losing your precious baby.

What I will say, however, is that sometimes it is better to know these things. It is a horrid time to find out that some friendships aren't built to last, but we all deserve to have friends who can walk with us in both good and bad times. If certain people can't handle the bad, they are better off not journeying life with us at all.

I do hope that you have also gained some new friends following having gone through loss. Some of the friends I made after losing my children are now more like family. The friendships are so deep because they were built through genuine connection and heartfelt sharing. If you haven't found new friends yet, keep seeking them out.

But it's not just loss that can change relationships, pregnancy can do this too.

Pregnancy can change friendships for the better or worse. So how can we make it be the former rather than the latter?

I have a few tips that may help:

- Firstly, try not to talk only about your pregnancy unless you are both pregnant at the same time. Remember that, to your friend, your pregnancy is just one topic of conversation. Just like you would find it tedious if they only talked about work, they may struggle if you talk about nothing but your pregnancy.
- Secondly, ensure you keep asking your friends about their lives and their plans. When you are pregnant, it can be hard to think of anything else, and at times that can come across as a person not being interested in anything other than their growing bump. Ensure it doesn't look like that, by staying present and engaged in your friends' lives.
- Thirdly, try to include any friends who want to be involved in your pregnancy. Share with them the good news and let them walk this path with you. It is easy to shut yourself off from the world when you are facing challenges, and that can mean our friends feel abandoned. Try to let them journey this with you, and

hopefully you will have an even stronger friendship when your baby arrives in your arms.

Today I am grateful for

```
┌─────────────────────────────────────────────┐
│                                             │
│                                             │
│                                             │
└─────────────────────────────────────────────┘
```

DAY 5

Journalling your pregnancy

What gestation is your baby today? _____

How big are they? _____

What symptoms are you now feeling?

```
┌─────────────────────────────────────────────┐
│                                             │
│                                             │
│                                             │
└─────────────────────────────────────────────┘
```

What do you want to remember about how you are feeling or what you are experiencing?

```
┌─────────────────────────────────────────────┐
│                                             │
│                                             │
│                                             │
│                                             │
│                                             │
│                                             │
└─────────────────────────────────────────────┘
```

The love I carry for you makes me braver,
for now I carry your sword and mine.

ZOË CLARK-COATES

Today I am grateful for

DAY 6

Support – When loss has removed your confidence in gut feelings and instinct

Loss of self-confidence is a horrible side effect of baby loss, and many people suffer from it. For some, it happens as their world has been tipped upside down and they don't even know which way is up anymore. For others it occurs because something they truly believed would be the case turns out not to be.

Their belief system has been shattered, and it is as if their internal compass is then destroyed.

Often people say they feel that they have regressed emotionally and they feel almost childlike; this can make them yearn to be taken care of and they relish the thought of others making decisions for them. I would encourage you to navigate this feeling of vulnerability by starting to make little decisions, such as deciding what's for dinner, or where to visit at the weekend – things that are relatively simple and carry little consequence, so your confidence can be rebuilt over a period of time. The greater the number of small choices you can make, the stronger your confidence will be when you need to make more monumental decisions.

Regarding your gut instincts being disarmed, again this is normal. It is very hard to deal with no longer knowing the difference between a gut feeling and an irrational fear.

Many are scared to ignore the feeling of worry in case it's their gut instinct alerting them to an issue, but they are also concerned that it could just be panic pushing them and not instinct at all. Please talk about this with your doctor or midwife and also your partner or a friend. Explain that your 'go-to' instinct at the moment is worry, so you have lost faith in your ability to gauge situations well. Ask for their help in knowing when to act and when to relax.

Today I am grateful for

DAY 7

Journal

If you could change something about your life, what would you change and why? How would this benefit your life and is it possible to actually do it?

What do you love to do? Do you spend enough time doing it? If not, can you create more time in your schedule so you can do it more?

I used to think my biggest flaw
was feeling it all so deeply,
now I acknowledge that it's one
of my greatest strengths.
What could have broken me
made me stronger . . .
And those valleys that were
created in my soul from
experiencing loss are now
vessels that can
hold deeper levels of joy.

ZOË CLARK-COATES

Today I am grateful for

WEEK 8

• •

DAY 1

Support – Feeling ill, and not wanting to complain as you believe you should only feel gratitude

This is such a tough feeling to negotiate. When I was pregnant with Brontë, I was very ill from four weeks of pregnancy until delivery, and I know I was burdened by this. How can you complain about the symptoms of pregnancy when all you wanted to be was pregnant? How can you complain about feeling nauseous when last year you were begging for pregnancy symptoms to take hold? We can end up constantly berating ourselves for not feeling permanently grateful. Let me assure you that feeling ill (or anxious, etc.) in no way removes your gratitude for being pregnant and growing a longed-for child. One feeling does not erase another, and if anyone tells you it does, they are wrong. If you are suffering, it is OK to say so, my friend.

Today I am grateful for

DAY 2

Task

Spend time today creating your own music playlist. Think of creating a list to listen to when you want to be inspired or distracted.

Today I am grateful for

DAY 3

EXPERT OPINION

Dr Jessica Farren MA, MBBS, MRCOG, PhD, OBGYN

Why do some people have pregnancy symptoms and others don't?

This is a question that doctors have been trying to answer for a long time! If we could understand this, then we might understand better why some women get very severe and unpleasant symptoms – such as hyperemesis (severe nausea and vomiting in pregnancy) – and be better able to find a solution.

What we do know is that women who have very strong symptoms are more likely to have strong symptoms in a subsequent pregnancy and that women carrying twin pregnancies are also more likely to have symptoms that are difficult to manage. However, symptoms don't seem to correlate very well with the amount of pregnancy hormone found on any blood tests.

Breast tenderness and growth is very variable depending on the size and makeup of your breasts. Just like there is a huge variation in whether women experience breast pain and tenderness with their menstrual cycle, the way the breasts respond to the rapidly changing hormone levels in early pregnancy also varies enormously.

Some women even experience significant differences from one healthy pregnancy to the next – so your symptoms in one pregnancy may not be a predictor of your symptoms in another. This, too, is nothing to worry about.

If pregnancy symptoms suddenly stop, does that mean there is a problem?

Certainly not. It is widely recognised that pregnancy symptoms come and go – and can change significantly from one day to the next, or one hour to the next.

Some women who have pregnancy losses anecdotally remember feeling that sickness, breast tenderness and tiredness lessened around the time the pregnancy stopped growing – and this understandably makes them anxious if they notice a change in a subsequent pregnancy. However, most 'sudden' changes change back just as suddenly – and you have to remember that the brain is very capable of playing tricks on you when you are anxious, and making you feel as though the symptoms have completely disappeared, only for them to return with a bang when you've had some reassurance.

If your concerns persist over a few days, you should definitely ask for a scan for reassurance, to put your mind at rest.

Is there anything you can do to help pregnancy nausea/sickness?

Women often find that nausea is worse when they are hungry. For this reason, it is often a good idea to keep snacks with you at all times – and have something to nibble on when the sickness comes. It's worth experimenting a little bit with what appeals, and what works for you – but crackers, bananas or dry toast are sensible options to try.

Ginger has a good reputation, and has been found in some studies to make symptoms better – but many women find the intense flavour makes their symptoms worse (and get very fed up of being offered ginger biscuits by well-meaning friends).

Some women find very cold things more appealing when they feel nauseous – crushed ice can be a great way to keep well hydrated. Some women also find that cold soft drinks, such as cola, with a spoonful of sugar to take the fizz out (but beware – this can cause it to bubble over!) can be just what they fancy, and a good way to get some calories and energy when it is really hard to keep anything down.

It's usually best to avoid spicy or acidic food or drink such as curry, pineapple or orange juice, as these can make an already sore lining to your stomach even more irritated.

If symptoms are difficult to manage, it is worth getting some anti-sickness medications prescribed. There are lots of different options, and they all have been used extensively in pregnancy and have been shown to be safe. If your symptoms are severe and it becomes difficult to keep anything down, you may need to go to the hospital for intravenous rehydration, where fluid is replaced through a small needle into a vein, and anti-sickness medication. Sometimes a course of steroids is required.

It is important to say that experiencing sickness does not represent any risks to your pregnancy. It does not increase your risk of miscarriage. Women understandably get concerned that they need to be eating as healthily as possible in the early stages of pregnancy, and panic if they're struggling to eat well – but the reality is that the tiny pregnancy is more than capable of stealing all its minimal requirements to grow from your existing stores. We do suggest that you continue to try to take folic acid (400mcg once each day, to minimise the risk of conditions that affect the development of the baby's spine) – but if you are struggling to take large multivitamin tablets, you may find the tiny tablets of only folic acid are easier to tolerate.

It's also worth saying that persistent nausea and/or vomiting in early pregnancy can often understandably make women feel very low in mood. This can be a confusing emotion – especially when you feel you 'should' be happy to be showing signs of a healthy pregnancy. But it is important to be kind to yourself during these times. Please be reassured that the sickness does usually pass in the second trimester (though often not as early as the 12 weeks people are led to expect) – and women often find their mood improves as the sickness does.

Today I am grateful for

DAY 4

Support – Feeling guilty about being pregnant when others have just lost

When you have felt that pain of hearing another pregnancy announcement after your own loss, you want to protect others from feeling those emotions. Sadly, just like you couldn't be protected, you can't protect others.

That said, of course you can be sensitive in how you deliver your news and be wise about how you broadcast your pregnancy. I would like to mention that not everyone is affected by pregnancy announcements; I wasn't. I was never triggered by friends getting pregnant, or by seeing bumps everywhere; in fact, they brought me hope that happy endings were possible. All I would say is be sensitive, and ask people how they are feeling rather than presume.

If you are concerned about how a grieving friend might take your announcement, I would advise telling them privately, before you make anything public. Ideally, email them or send a text, rather than doing it face to face. I encourage this, rather than breaking the news in person, as it allows people to compose themselves and respond in a way they are happy with. It can be tricky to pull off an Oscar-winning performance with no warning. It also means that if they are upset, they can gather themselves before responding.

I would never advise including any presumptions about their feelings in your message, such as, 'I know this is going to hurt you, but I wanted to let you know I am pregnant.' Firstly, you don't know it will upset them, and secondly, by highlighting their reaction, you may be encouraging them to feel shame or embarrassment. Choose your words carefully, perhaps something as simple as, 'I wanted to tell you privately that we are having a baby. We love you and support you and totally understand if you wish to or don't want to acknowledge the pregnancy. It is fine not to message us back, but we wanted you to know.' A message like this removes any pressure the friend may feel and they can then respond or not respond to the message.

The fear of upsetting friends who have lost a baby can run so deep that, at times, people try to avoid seeing these friends while they are sporting a pregnancy bump. This kind of avoidance – however well-intended – can cause more harm and emotional upset. I strongly advise you to be mindful of this and be guided by those friends, and ask them to set the ground rules.

Today I am grateful for

DAY 5

Journalling your pregnancy

What gestation is your baby today? _____

How big are they? _____

What symptoms are you now feeling?

What do you want to remember about how you are feeling
or what you are experiencing?

> As the seasons change so does our grief.
> This is how nature shows us that the beauty of life
> is that it goes on.
>
> ZOË CLARK-COATES

Today I am grateful for

DAY 6

Support – Loving pregnancy or hating pregnancy

It is OK to love your pregnancy and it's equally fine to hate
it, even if you have longed to be pregnant. Most people will

love parts and hate parts. You can despise pregnancy and adore your baby, just like you can loathe your job but delight in earning money. The pressure to feel a certain way is one of the most significant issues here, as expectation can bring with it feelings of shame and failure. My pregnancies with my two daughters, whom I am blessed to raise, were poles apart. I experienced diverse emotions while pregnant with them both. One pregnancy was way more peaceful than the other, and when you are terrified 24/7 that's an understandably hard journey to enjoy – but I always adored the fact I was growing a baby. I loved that special feeling of protecting my child. So the bottom line is you have to just go with it, you feel what you feel, and you feel it guilt-free!

Today I am grateful for

DAY 7

Journal

List five people, situations or life lessons you are grateful for.

1 _____

2 _____

3 _____

4 _____

5 _____

What five goals do you have for the future? Maybe they are goals for your career, for your family? Perhaps you want to travel to certain parts of the world? Or maybe they are more personal goals, to have counselling to address a traumatic situation?

1 _____

2 _____

3 _____

4 _____

5 _____

· ·

When you allow yourself to believe
that a good thing may happen
you are allowing those seeds of faith
to bloom into hope.

· · · · · · · · · · · · ZOË CLARK-COATES · · · · · · · · · · · · ·

Today I am grateful for

WEEK 9

• •

DAY 1

Support – Scans

Time goes so slowly when you are waiting for a scan. In an ideal world a scan should be an exciting event to look forward to, but, post-loss, the anticipation can be filled with dread.

If this is your first-ever scan, what can you expect?

In the UK you are usually offered two scans, one around 12 weeks' gestation and one around 20 weeks. This differs in other countries.

Ideally, you should go to a scan with a full bladder as this gives the sonographer the best chance of capturing excellent images, but if this isn't possible don't panic too much, as modern equipment makes this less of a necessity.

Please tell the person who is doing your scan about your history with loss. Tell them you would appreciate their reassurance and them talking you through the scan as it's being done.

During the appointment, you will be asked to lie on a bed and gel will be applied to your stomach. The sonographer will then press the wand into the gel and gently move it over your belly. At times they will use some pressure, but this is normal and nothing to worry about.

It may take them a little time to locate your baby, and its heartbeat, as babies have a knack of playing hide-and-seek at the worst possible times. It is totally normal to try to read the face of the person conducting the scan, but I promise you they often show very little expression and stay fairly silent as they have to focus on their task.

Once they have found the baby, they will then start measuring and recording all dimensions. These measurements are logged onto the computer, which tells the sonographer how the baby measures against other babies of the same gestation. The baby will be given a range on a centile chart. From this, you will be able to see if your baby measures similarly to others of the same gestation, and this information helps your medical team assess whether your baby appears to be growing normally. It is important to remember that all babies grow at different rates. Some have big growth spurts outside of what would be construed as standard. So do not panic if your baby shows as being small for its gestation, just talk with your medical team to get the reassurance you need. Once your scan is completed, they will wipe off the remaining gel from your stomach, and the scan will be over.

The 20-week scan is longer in duration as it involves a lot more checks of the baby. Your baby's heart will be thoroughly checked, as well as all the other organs. Bones are measured and so much more. They will also be checking that your placenta looks healthy and that blood flow to and from it is steady.

If your medical team have any concerns, or if they are closely monitoring you, you may be offered further scans. For many post-loss parents, these extra scans can provide vital peace of mind and are generally welcomed by all.

Transvaginal scans – these internal scans were once the norm. In layman's terms, the sonographer puts a condom over a scanning wand (that sounds far more magical than it is!), and inserts it into your vagina. Thanks to advanced scanning techniques, and more high-tech equipment being developed, these are needed less often now, so many people go through an entire pregnancy without having to have an internal scan.

At times, however, an internal scan may be required, especially if it is a scan being done at a very early gestation to investigate bleeding or to see if a heartbeat is present. A lot of people fear this type of scan, but let me reassure you that it isn't at all painful, and it's over very quickly.

The first time I needed to have a transvaginal scan, I was so worried that my lovely consultant suggested my husband Andy conduct the scan, while the doctor shouted instructions through the curtains. I still laugh a lot about this, especially the bit when we were exiting the clinic, and Andy turned to me and said, 'I have to add this newly discovered skill to my CV.' Anyway, there is nothing to fear. If you are nervous, just let your sonographer know, and ask them to explain what they are doing.

Today I am grateful for

DAY 2

Task

Find a poem that accurately describes how you are feeling at the moment. If you can't find one, or if you prefer, write your own.

Today I am grateful for

DAY 3

Becky's Story

Like every other mother who longs for a baby, there was nothing quite like my first positive pregnancy test. Unlike some of my friends at the time, I was grateful that I had fallen pregnant fairly quickly and easily, as I couldn't have been more ready to start a family. I had wanted to become a mum for a couple of years, but we were living in a small flat in London and couldn't see how we would make ends meet if I wasn't working. However, we finally reached a point of realising we had to stop fearing and just go for it. Somehow it would all work out.

The elation of realising a baby was growing inside me was overwhelming. I remember the first thing I did was to sit down at the piano and sing, expressing my joy and wonder at this new life. My husband, Nick, was equally delighted and we spent time researching every detail of our child's early development, buying books and endlessly talking about names.

Due to there being a culture of not telling people you were pregnant until 12 weeks, that's what we did. We literally didn't tell a soul.

Three more weeks passed, and everything in my

body was changing. I was exhausted and hormonal; but very excited about what was coming. And then one day, I went shopping with my mum, and the most terrible pains started. I began bleeding, and the pain got so bad I nearly fainted on the street. My mum had to call an ambulance to get me to the hospital. One of the hardest things was sitting on a bench on the high street explaining to my mum through tears that I was pregnant but clearly miscarrying. It was a confusing conversation – the last thing I needed at this point. Note to self: if I'm ever pregnant again, tell those closest to me straight away.

The scan showed that the baby had died. I was incredibly sad and shocked. A nurse said to me that I should wait several months for my body to return to normal before trying for a baby again, which was a double whammy! Even as I was miscarrying, I was utterly desperate to get pregnant again. I didn't share that with her, as I somehow felt ashamed it wasn't the 'right' thing to want. But the joy of carrying my first baby, as short-lived as it was, had been so immense that I felt empty and longed for that joy again. I learnt my first lesson about miscarriage there in the hospital – people will have all manner of views and advice on what you should or shouldn't do or feel about miscarriage, and it's important to give yourself the freedom to do exactly what works for you. Some women may have felt the need to wait a while, take stock and recover. I needed to crack on. Both are OK.

Amazingly, I was able to conceive again quickly, but the joy I had anticipated and longed for was absent this time around. I think the hardest part of miscarrying your first child is that it robs you of future joy in early pregnancy. Yes, I was delighted to find out I was expecting again, but this time fear set in. What if I would never carry a baby to full term? What if there's a bigger problem with my womb? What if it happens again? However, I had also learnt that I didn't want to make it a big secret this time around. We told my parents and some close friends immediately.

I have a strong Christian faith, and for me, one of the biggest comforts was that I knew my friends were praying for the baby and me. I remember one day at work I began to get pains. I realise now that they were probably growing and stretching pains, which can be remarkably similar to the feeling of low-level contractions, but at the time I was terrified it was happening again. I went outside and called my friend. She prayed with me over the phone, and I felt strengthened and supported.

For me, getting further on in my pregnancy this time was very significant. After my first scan, I was able to finally relax and enjoy the pregnancy, confident that all would be well. One of the good consequences of losing a baby through miscarriage is that despite the inevitable fear of it happening again, there is also a deeper appreciation that arises. I did not take this pregnancy for granted. I think it knocked out of me any sense of entitlement. I marvelled at the life being formed within me and realised that I am not in control.

I went on to have two beautiful children, but some time later, I fell pregnant again, and sadly I lost this baby in an early miscarriage.

This loss was a very different experience for me from my first miscarriage. This time, I didn't carry the fear of 'What if I never manage to carry a baby?' I knew my body could do that. But with this loss, I knew far more keenly the love I would have had for this baby. I already adored my two children, and in a sense, I knew far more now what I was missing. There was also a different kind of shock that went with this miscarriage. Having carried two children to full term, I think part of me assumed my body would go on doing that. I'd also had pregnancy symptoms and felt like everything was progressing normally, so the shock was greater. I learnt here that no two losses are ever the same. Both were a complicated mix of many feelings and meanings. The added stress of this second loss was that I had to have surgical management, and I found that day in the hospital very traumatic. I had to go alone as Nick had the two children, and I felt a sense of dread and loneliness all day.

I went on to have another two children. Following my second miscarriage, I had the familiar feelings of desperation to be pregnant again, plus the impending fear of another loss. By this stage in my life, I was talking much more openly about my miscarriages, and I found that people can be either extremely compassionate or very unhelpful.

As I navigated the lows of these losses, quite simply I just needed compassion and a listening ear. I got huge comfort from talking to friends who had been through it. I had to seek them out, though, as many older women I knew had been through the same thing but had never talked about it. One woman whom I knew well had had a miscarriage and even held a small funeral service for her baby, but I'd had no idea. As I shared my story with her, she opened up, and we found a real connection. The culture is definitely changing, even in the past decade, and with charities like sayinggoodbye.org raising the profile of baby loss, I am finally hearing more and more women talking about their experience of losing a child.

My final reflection now, as a mum of six who gets to

raise only four, is that without my two losses, I wouldn't have a single one of my current children. The children who didn't make it into this world have somehow made way for these other beautiful children to survive and make it through. It's a strange but amazing thing. And for me, it's the only thing that actually helps me to make any sense of the pain I went through.

Today I am grateful for

DAY 4

Support – Should I have private scans?

This is a personal decision and not one I can advise on. Did I have them? Yes, I did. For me, they brought me a great deal of reassurance. I always paid for an early scan at around five weeks to ensure things were in the right place, and then I had regular scans after that. If you do decide to go to a private clinic, I would always advise the following:

1. Ensure it's a reputable clinic – i.e. run by midwives, OBGYNs (doctors specialising in obstetrics and gynaecology) or trained sonographers. There are so many clinics that are run by untrained people, and this may add to your worry, or not help alleviate it.
2. Ask if you will be given photos or a DVD of the scan to keep.

3. If they advise you to have an additional scan, do you have to pay again or will they do it for free?

How do you request additional NHS scans if you are worried?

Well, it all depends on what you are worried about. If you have had any bleeding or other physical symptoms, your midwife or GP should be able and willing to request a scan for you. If you need a scan due to worry, this will be at the discretion of your medical team, so talk with them.

Today I am grateful for

DAY 5

Journalling your pregnancy

What gestation is your baby today? _____

How big are they? _____

What symptoms are you now feeling?

What do you want to remember about how you are feeling or what you are experiencing?

> If you choose not to grieve, you are choosing not to love as the two are irrevocably tied together.
>
> ZOË CLARK-COATES

Today I am grateful for

DAY 6

Support – How to tell people you are expecting

I think most people are very aware that I don't believe in the 12-week rule 'not to tell anyone you are pregnant until after your first scan', as I believe this is a not-so-subtle message to keep people silent if they encounter loss. I hold the view that people should feel the freedom to tell people they are pregnant as soon as they feel ready to do so.

So when people are ready, how should they share their special news?

I think once you have encountered loss first-hand you are so mindful of the pain pregnancy announcements can have on those who are having fertility issues, or who have lost a baby, and you never want your baby announcement to cause pain in someone else's life. Sadly, there is no way to prevent all suffering, and, as I mentioned earlier, the only thing you can do is be sensitive in how you announce your pregnancy.

- My first piece of advice would be to avoid social media announcements altogether. You cannot control who sees these, and you have no clue when people may see your news, so it is much better to tell people in written messages (text, email, letter), as this gives them space to process your news before responding. If it's not possible to share your news in writing, ensure you tell people in private, whether that be over the phone, or face to face, so they don't need to contend with an audience.
- When you tell people, choose the language you use carefully. Be mindful that you won't know everyone's story; many people keep their losses and pain hidden.
- Tell your inner circle first, to avoid the people closest to you feeling hurt.
- Finally, try to prepare yourself for insensitive comments (such as, 'Now you will be able to put your loss behind you'). So many people say the wrong thing in the moment, and then regret it. I heard so many hurtful things when we told people we were expecting again, and while I know no one intended to cause us upset, they didn't think carefully about the words they used. So just be ready, and try to have buckets of grace on standby, as there is a good chance you will need them.

Today I am grateful for

[ ]

DAY 7

Journal

What would you tell 18-year-old you?

[ ]

'In the waiting'
This sacred period of time that most of us despise.
It's a time where our limits are tested,
our belief is questioned and the only thing that
can carry us through is hope.

ZOË CLARK-COATES

Today I am grateful for

[ ]

WEEK 10

• •

DAY 1

Support – Social media and pregnancy

I am sure like most people you have a love-hate relationship with social media. Whether it be Facebook, Instagram, Twitter or another social media platform, all of them have their positives and negatives.

Some prefer to stay away from them when pregnant, while for others they can be a lifeline, as they offer them a direct connection with the outside world without the need to even leave the comfort of their own home. Only you know whether using social media is a good or bad thing for you, and it is vital to properly consider where it helps you and where it may not.

One of the significant issues with social media is that people may offer unsolicited opinions and advice, and this can be trying at the best of times. I handle this by not posting anything on social media platforms unless I am ready to face the comments, and I can honestly say this has helped me avoid a host of unwanted advice. If I do want to share things on social media, I often choose my private Facebook page, and I then carefully select the audience that can see the post.

Another problem with social media is that nuance and context get stripped out of what is being said. People may also say or word things in ways they would not do in face-to-face conversations. It is easy to take offence, and it is easy to read between the lines (and see things that are not intended). If you feel vulnerable, it may be wise to avoid going on social media at all, as the last thing you need right now is personal upset or arguments.

If you do choose to use social media, remember that most of the platforms allow you to select the content you see. For instance, you can choose which posts by friends and family you see on Facebook. The same applies to Instagram and Twitter; you can follow people but hide or mute their content. This means you can stay connected (and not cause upset or offence) and still protect yourself from seeing things you would rather not see.

If you do use social media come find me on Facebook, Twitter and Instagram, as I post daily support messages for people who are struggling.

Today I am grateful for

DAY 2

Task

How would you describe pregnancy post-loss to someone who hasn't ever experienced it?

Today I am grateful for

DAY 3

Siobhan Abrahams BSc (Hons), Clin Dip Pharm, IP, lead pharmacist in an NHS Trust

What medications can a pregnant person take safely?

The safety of the use of medicines in pregnancy depends on several factors.

Background: testing of medicines

Some medicines have been around for a very long time, and so there is a lot of knowledge about the safety of the mother, baby and, in some cases, the babies of those babies. Drug companies tend to do research of drugs on young men, and it is only when the drugs are given to women who are pregnant that the effects are known. Most of the common medicines that you can buy from a pharmacy have been around a long time, paracetamol since the 1870s and ibuprofen since the 1950s, so have been through these testing cycles. Some of the newer medications do not have so much information about use in pregnancy, and so the drug companies tend to advise against use.

Medication for long-term conditions

Some medicines are unsafe in pregnancy, for example sodium valproate (Epilim), which is used in epilepsy or some mental

health conditions. It is important, if you are on long-term medication and you think that you may like to become pregnant, that you speak to your pharmacist or doctor about the safety of your medication before you start trying. It may be that your medication is absolutely fine in pregnancy or it may be that you can be changed onto another safer medication while pregnant. It may be that the doctors decide that the risk to your health of changing or stopping the medication would be greater than the risk to the baby and so would monitor you and baby while pregnant. This is the case with some mental health medication where it is important to keep you mentally stable and safe, and so consequently keeping the baby safe.

Many medicines differ in how safe they are depending on the trimester of the pregnancy as the baby develops. The ideal is not to use pharmacological methods (medicines) when pregnant, but sometimes it is necessary for both your well-being and that of the baby. Some medicines, for example ibuprofen, are now known to be relatively safe in the first two trimesters, but not in the third trimester. With a medication such as codeine or morphine, as you get closer to birth, it may cause difficulty with the baby's breathing. This can be monitored and managed, so it is not a reason to exclude taking the medication, just to be cautious.

What practical considerations should I remember?

When taking medications that you buy over the counter, for pain relief for example, then it is advised that you take the smallest successful dose for the shortest period of time. It is worth thinking too about how the side effects will affect your body. Some pain relief containing codeine can cause constipation, so you may need to take a laxative at the same time, and it is also important that you optimise your fluid and dietary intake. Joint pain may be relieved by wearing braces or applying heat pads. Always speak to your doctor, midwife or a pharmacist before taking any medication.

Where can I obtain further information?

Ask your local pharmacist or doctor for further information. If you want to do your own research I would suggest looking at medicinesinpregnancy.org (Bumps UK). This is one of the best resources for information about individual medicine use in pregnancy. The information is provided by the UK Teratology Information Service (UKTIS). UKTIS is a not-for-profit organisation funded by Public Health England on behalf of the UK Health Departments. It provides information on the safety of the individual medications, including the risk of miscarriage, stillbirth, pre-term birth, congenital disabilities, low birth weight and need for extra monitoring as well as any other health issues they may cause. There are individual leaflets for the different medicines that are accessible from the website.

Today I am grateful for

DAY 4

Support – Envy of others having an easier pregnancy, or being able to think positively

It is hard when you see someone else having what looks like an easy time when it feels like you are going through hell. What I am always mindful of, however, is that some people are just excellent at making things look easy, and it doesn't mean that is actually how it is.

That said, some lucky people do get pregnant easily, have super-straightforward pregnancies and then easy deliveries, and others don't. For some in the latter category, the comparison can become a real issue.

I am a big believer in trying not to be envious of anyone, and I make a conscious choice to be happy for people, even if things don't appear to be fair. The only small bit of advice I can offer is that the choice to focus on happiness can eventually seep deeper into your soul. I always hear people say you can choose to forgive, and eventually your heart agrees, and I think a similar thing applies when talking about finding joy in another's happiness.

If you do feel jealous, please don't let this completely understandable emotion bring you additional worry or anxiety. Just acknowledge this is how you feel right now, and acknowledge there is a very good reason why you feel it. Let any shame go, and forgive yourself if you are feeling guilty. None of the emotions you feel define you; they are purely transient feelings that will pass over time.

Today I am grateful for

DAY 5

Journalling your pregnancy

What gestation is your baby today? _____

How big are they? _____

What symptoms are you now feeling?

What do you want to remember about how you are feeling or what you are experiencing?

. . . .

I never knew if I believed in love at first sight,
but the fact that I love you before
I have even seen you
shows me it must be real.

. . . . ZOË CLARK-COATES . . . .

Today I am grateful for

> ```
> 
> 
> 
> ```

DAY 6

Support – Loo terror

Something I never knew existed until I had lost my first baby.
So what is 'loo terror'?

It is the name I came up with for the fear that develops post-loss. When you feel utterly terrified of going to the loo while pregnant (or even when you aren't pregnant) just in case you see blood in your underwear, on loo roll or in the toilet itself. Because of the terror of seeing red, people then either avoid using the loo or can become obsessive about going to the bathroom to check for any signs of blood.

If you haven't ever experienced this, it's probably hard to grasp the magnitude of it, but it can be pretty debilitating for those who suffer with it acutely. It can affect people's work life, home life and rob them of vital and much-needed sleep.

I remember well how I would have to work up the courage to go to the loo. At night I would occasionally summon the courage to give myself time off from checking, and would use the bathroom in the dark so that I couldn't check anything.

At its worst, people drink less fluid so they can reduce the number of loo visits. They avoid going out to places in case they see red in public restrooms, and they make themselves sore from constant wiping. The emotional effect is also significant as people feel they are living on a knife-edge, in a constant state of anxiety. This then heightens their fight-or-flight response.

If you are experiencing or have experienced this, please know you are not alone. This is very common after loss.

So what tips can I offer to help navigate it?

1. Talk with a professional, or at the very least your partner or a friend, about your feelings. Some find they need therapy to be free of this fear, while others find freedom over time.
2. Practise your relaxation exercises before going to the loo and even while on the loo. Reassure yourself that all is well.
3. I found avoiding wearing red underwear or clothes helped me, as any rogue red threads or fluff sent me into a panic.
4. Be careful what loo roll you use. Anyone who has lived with this fear will tell you recycled loo paper or cheaper varieties can often have multicoloured specks in the paper, and when you encounter a red dot, it can make you want to pass out.

Today I am grateful for

DAY 7

Journal

List five positive changes you would like to make in your life.

1 _____

2 _____

3 _____

4 _____

5 _____

• •

It is in the waiting
that we must hold
on to hope.

• • • • • • • • • • • • • ZOË CLARK-COATES • • • • • • • • • • • • • •

Today I am grateful for

WEEK 11

• •

DAY 1

Support – Relationships with your medical team

The relationship you have with your doctor, or OBGYN, and midwife is vital post-loss as they can offer you crucial support and advice. It is, of course, just as important pre-loss, but as this book is only focused on pregnancy post-loss I am concentrating on the relationship with them now you are pregnant again.

I don't know about you, but I find it so hard to complain about poor service or treatment, and this definitely extends to when I am offered inferior or substandard medical care. It feels awkward and like I am making a fuss if I ask to see someone else or request a second opinion. I will say to you what I have to say to myself when it comes to good care: you have to just overcome this desire to conform and not complain. You have to boldly ask (and even demand) the excellent care you and your baby deserve.

Great care doesn't just mean proper medical treatment, it also involves receiving good mental health support, so if you aren't getting it, speak up and ask for someone else to take over your care.

Today I am grateful for

DAY 2

Task

How do you feel you have changed since going through loss? And how do you feel pregnancy has already changed you?

Today I am grateful for

DAY 3

Nicola's Story

A positive pregnancy test. In the light of our previous loss, I thought I'd be relieved, happy, reinvigorated. In fact, I was deeply sad. With the positive result came a sense of finality to the pregnancy I was supposed to be still living with. Although I was fully aware we had lost our baby months earlier, now there really was no way there had been a mistake. Foolish, I know. I cried when I told my husband about the new pregnancy, because the emotions were too strong and too confusing. I had to let out some tears and groans, praying that this sadness wouldn't affect the new life I was holding, and feeling guilty for not celebrating this baby. But the celebration could wait, I was confident of that.

I remember feeling embarrassed to tell people who knew about our loss that we were now expecting again, because in my mind they might assume that I was, therefore, 'over it' – not true. Or what if they assumed that we'd planned a pregnancy as soon as possible? As if becoming pregnant again was a 'fix' – it isn't. I worried they would think I hadn't valued the lost life enough, as though there was an acceptable period of time to mourn before you become pregnant again (nine months maybe) and we hadn't met that.

Or maybe – and the thought I battled the most – they would silently let out a sigh of relief that they no longer had to think of me as someone who was grieving. Or perhaps they'd feel they didn't have to tiptoe around me. Because now I was pregnant, so all was fine. It put an end to all the miscarriage chat. And all of these thoughts, often unhelpful and unjustified, were really hard to manage.

I remember finding it very odd when people asked questions like, 'Will you find out the gender?', as though I might be preoccupied with that outcome. I wasn't. I was preoccupied with this baby surviving.

I remember people asking, 'Have you been trying?' What a personal question! So I gave a personal answer: 'Actually we had a miscarriage earlier in the year, and we're still working that out.' I wasn't trying to cut people down to size, but I had wanted to be open about our miscarriage after being so shocked by the statistics.

Once I started to tell people, I was amazed at how many quiet, but strong voices responded with, 'Yeah, we've been through that too.' It really highlighted to me how little we talk about baby loss as a society.

I was five months pregnant when we hit the due date of the baby we had lost. A friend sent a 'thinking of you' card, which I was very touched by. She was the only one who acknowledged the due date. I wondered why some didn't check in but suspected all was forgotten with my emerging bump.

The hardest challenge was going to the toilet without checking for bleeding. I found this the most difficult thought pattern to shake because I was alone for that moment – it was all on me. I wanted someone to escort me to the loo and chat to me about *Bake Off*. Or anything that would distract me. But, thank goodness, it did get easier. And throughout the remainder of the pregnancy, I chose to live in hope.

I chose to reject fear. I would not have this pregnancy stolen from me by my thoughts. It doesn't quite make sense to me how I was able to do that. But I can honestly say that I managed to separate the two pregnancies and make a rightful acknowledgement of each, and distinction between the two. This is necessary as every pregnancy is unique, and brings its own challenges and surprises. Just as every baby does, and our boy's time did come to be celebrated. He has a double measure of joy – of that I am sure.

Today I am grateful for

DAY 4

Support – Wanting your medical team to be aware of a previous loss

Some people use a sticker on their pregnancy notes to alert the medical staff to a previous loss. I purely wrote it onto my notes. This meant everyone I saw who looked at my notes was instantly aware of my past losses and they were able to adapt the language they used; for instance, 'I can see this is not your first baby, as you have sadly lost children.'

Ensuring my notes stated what had happened meant I didn't need to keep saying the same thing over and over, which would otherwise have been a potential trigger for me when I was already anxious. If you want to tell your story in full, I would advise taking some time to type up your experience. Then you can print it out and put it in your notes. At the top of your story write: *I would appreciate you reading this if you are involved in my medical care during pregnancy.* Doing this can truly change the care you receive, and just knowing you don't need to keep telling your story makes appointments far less stressful.

Today I am grateful for

[ ]

DAY 5

Journalling your pregnancy

What gestation is your baby today? _____

How big are they? _____

What symptoms are you now feeling?

[ ]

What do you want to remember about how you are feeling or what you are experiencing?

[ ]

I have found one of the main panic triggers for
people is an expectation from others.
That can be an expectation of doing something,
being somewhere, looking a certain way.
If a person feels trapped into doing a
certain action, the result is often panic.

ZOË CLARK-COATES

Today I am grateful for

DAY 6

Support – Guilt

I think guilt accompanies everything connected to being a
parent; why I don't know, but it does. We feel we should
turn into superheroes when we have created a child, whether
they live or not. We feel we should suddenly be aware of
everything. Know every answer. Avoid every hazard. The
truth is, that isn't how life works. We are just all flawed
humans trying to do the best we can. We can only act on
the information we are aware of, and it's simply not possible
to know everything, even if we became a doctor or took a
master's degree in child development.

So give yourself a break, and be kind to yourself. Sometimes
we know the answers; sometimes we don't. Sometimes we do
the right thing; sometimes we do the wrong thing. All we can
do is the best we can at that moment.

Today I am grateful for

[ ]

DAY 7

Journal

Name five friends and write in the box what five special gifts they bring to your life.

1 _____

You give me

[ ]

2 _____

You give me

[ ]

3 _____

You give me

[ ]

4 _____

> You give me

5 _____

> You give me

. . . .

Hope is the ultimate guide
as it always knows
the way.

. . . . ZOË CLARK-COATES . . . .

Today I am grateful for

WEEK 12

DAY 1

Support – Fear of not bonding with the new baby

We all hear so much about bonding and this magical experience that takes place at birth, and I think most mothers will tell you they have a little, or a lot of, panic about this. It is hard not to think, 'What if bonding doesn't happen to me?' or, 'What if I look at my little one and feel nothing?' One worry quickly leads to another, and before you know it, you imagine yourself staring down at your newborn feeling nothing for them, and you can feel fear gripping you.

So let's look at this logically – could this happen?

Yes, of course, it could. We all know it is a possibility, and that is why we worry about it. We are fully aware there are times when this happens, as we read stories about it in the press. However, even if the bonding doesn't take place immediately, it is often just a delay in the process, and over subsequent weeks and months, those feelings will develop.

For the majority of people, then, the bonding feelings do appear, or perhaps they were always there from the moment you discovered your little one was growing within. What I can promise you is this – fearing a lack of bonding won't help you, and worrying won't change a thing. Most of you will bond deeply with your babies within days of their arrival, and you will look back at this worry you carried and laugh, as you will love your child more than life itself.

So try to relax, and permit yourself to feel anything and everything. Once you have released yourself from all pressure to feel a certain way, it makes the journey a lot more enjoyable.

Today I am grateful for

DAY 2

Task

Draw a picture or write a quote about how you are feeling right now. It is OK to feel anything, happiness, sadness – all emotions are valid.

Today I am grateful for

DAY 3

Dr Jacque Gerrard MBE, Midwife Consultant and former Director for England at the Royal College of Midwives

Are there any ways to help prevent baby loss?

Healthcare professionals, including midwives, do all that they can to support and advise women to help them have a healthy pregnancy. The government has published Safer Maternity Care *which aims to improve outcomes.*

NHS England advises the following:
- *Pre-conception: Take a daily folic acid supplement up until 12 weeks of pregnancy*
- *Stop smoking*
- *Cut out or down on alcohol*
- *Keep to a healthy weight*
- *Take moderate exercise*
- *Discuss prescription medications with your midwife or GP*
- *Get flu and whooping cough vaccinations*
- *If you have a long-term condition such as epilepsy or diabetes, then do not stop taking the medication but discuss this with the doctor*
- *Attend antenatal care clinics with a midwife*

How do you get more, or better, support from your midwife when you are nervous?

A trusting relationship must develop between the woman and the midwife. Hopefully, with the continuity of carer models being implemented via the Better Births policy across

---

England, *care will get better, and outcomes for mothers and babies will improve. A strong relationship will develop between the mother and the midwife within this model of care. The woman will then find it comfortable to share her anxieties and concerns, and the midwife can then better support and reassure her.*

Why do you get period-like pains when pregnant?

This period-like pain is known as Braxton Hicks contractions, where the womb contracts and relaxes, preparing the body for labour. They should not be painful but they are mildly uncomfortable. They are normal, and most women experience them during the second and third trimester. Women will notice that the abdomen tenses then relaxes. This happens intermittently and can last for some hours but then disappear, returning at another time. If the contractions develop into stronger pain, then the woman must contact a midwife or attend the labour ward for a check-up.

Is it OK to exercise when pregnant?

Yes. The chief medical officers in the UK advise healthy women with no complications in pregnancy to have 150 minutes of moderate exercise per week.

Today I am grateful for

DAY 4

Support – The 12-week rule

Anyone who follows my work or sayinggoodbye.org will know I am a massive believer in breaking the 12-week rule of not telling anyone you are pregnant until you have had your first scan, and I am sure I will mention it in this book multiple times, as it is such a bugbear of mine. This commonly discussed rule is a not-so-indirect way of telling people not to tell anyone if they encounter loss, and it's probably one of the biggest reasons that baby loss has been such a taboo subject. It is tough to tell anyone you have lost a baby if they didn't even know you were expecting in the first place, and when you need support more than ever, it's beyond harmful.

Those first few weeks of pregnancy can also be incredibly challenging, both physically and mentally. If you haven't informed people that you are pregnant, that means you get zero support at a time when you need the troops to rally around you.

Sit down with your partner and discuss how you both feel about sharing your news. If you are on the same page, discuss who you should tell. Do you tell everyone straight away, or just your family and closest friends? There is no right or wrong here, it is purely down to your personal feelings.

Today I am grateful for

DAY 5

Journalling your pregnancy

What gestation is your baby today? _____

How big are they? _____

What symptoms are you now feeling?

What do you want to remember about how you are feeling or what you are experiencing?

· ·

Sometimes people may make you
feel it is selfish to grieve.
It isn't.

· · · · · · · · · · · · ZOË CLARK-COATES · · · · · · · · · · · ·

Today I am grateful for

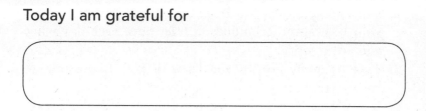

DAY 6

Support – Navigating work and pregnancy

Being pregnant at work can be complex at the best of times. When you couple that with being pregnant at work after a previous loss, it's doubly complicated. If you are struggling, please know I hear you, you are not alone in your feelings.

Whether you are trying to keep your pregnancy a secret at work, or whether your work colleagues know, try to take all the breaks you are entitled to and take moments where you can to go and relax. For some, having breaks is not part of their DNA: hands up, I am one of these, but when you are pregnant, you need to take breaks, as your body is already working so hard growing a human.

For some, having colleagues aware of their pregnancy makes work easier; for others it makes it harder as they would rather not focus on the baby at all in work hours. Only you know what is best for you, so you should handle it your way. If you are doing a job that is physically demanding you may want to let your line manager know you are expecting, just to ensure you and the baby are kept safe.

My top tips:

1. Try to tell at least one person you trust at work that you are pregnant, so you have someone to talk with if you are having a tough day.

2. Take all the breaks you are entitled to, and try to practise your relaxation techniques at least once each day while you are at work.
3. Take as many healthy snacks with you as possible, to ensure you keep your blood sugars stable.
4. If you have a desk job, ensure you take regular breaks and stretch your legs. If you sit still for too long, it can cause more aches and pains.
5. Work can offer you a great distraction, but try to maintain a good work-life balance, as rest time is important when you are pregnant.

Today I am grateful for

DAY 7

Journal

What makes you feel proud of yourself?

What was your most life-changing moment and how did it change you?

* *

This grief that you carry may not
diminish in weight,
but the muscles you have to carry it
will get stronger and stronger.

* * * * * * * * * * * * ZOË CLARK-COATES * * * * * * * * * * * *

Today I am grateful for

WEEK 13

DAY 1

Support – Taking photos

I didn't take enough photos. This is hands down one of my biggest pregnancy regrets, both with the babies who ran ahead, and the babies who got to stay. I so wish I had photos of every pregnancy bump at every stage. There is no way I can rewind time and capture those images, so let me encourage you to take as many pictures as you can. Every angle, flattering, unflattering, who cares! One day you will so appreciate having those images to look back on, as this is one of the most beautiful seasons of your life. Before you know it, this pregnancy will just be a memory, and you will be looking down at your newborn – so take the photos. Take ones of your bump, of your face, of you and your partner – take them all. This is your season of growth, so cherish it and capture it.

Today I am grateful for

DAY 2

Task

What film makes you laugh the most? Rewatch it. Then look for a new film that will make you smile and watch that. Sometimes we need to escape life, and for many watching movies helps them do just this. It's good for the mind to have times to stop thinking and just relax – try to do this as often as you can.

Today I am grateful for

DAY 3

Becki's Story

Our baby journey began, like most people's, full of hopeful anticipation of what was to come. We'd naïvely assumed that now we had decided to start having children, it would happen quickly and would go according to plan. I mean, how could there be this many people in the world if it wasn't easy? We couldn't have been more wrong.

After months (that seemed like years) of trying with no luck, I finally had a positive pregnancy test, and we were elated! We called our immediate family to share the news straight away and started dreaming of the future. However, those hopes and dreams came crashing down when I started to bleed. It started as spotting but got progressively heavier over the next few days until I lost the baby.

More torturous months crept by and life became a rollercoaster of emotions split into two-week increments – two weeks until I ovulated, then two weeks until I could take a test which always came back negative. At last, eight months after our miscarriage, I had another positive pregnancy test and all the hopeful anticipation came flooding back. Sadly, the excitement rapidly turned to despair when I started to bleed again and, just like before, we lost the baby early in the pregnancy.

It was the start of a new year, and with two baby losses and two years of trying unsuccessfully to start a family, I was losing hope fast. I was emotionally exhausted from the relentless tennis match between hope and disappointment. I felt broken and shamefully defective, surrounded by perfectly functioning fruitful women who were having babies left, right and centre. I was tired of battling with feelings of jealousy when yet another pregnancy was announced and the guilt and shame that swiftly followed because I selfishly couldn't feel joy for others.

We were now under the care of a fertility doctor who had determined that we had 'unexplained infertility'. This was both a blessing and a curse. I was very grateful that neither my husband nor I had any obvious issues, but without a cause, there was no clear way forward. Our doctor had suggested we wait until my next period arrived and then we could begin looking at doing a tracked cycle – the first of several options we could try.

I waited for the inevitable period bleeding, but it didn't arrive as expected. Unwilling to let myself get carried away, I assumed that I had miscalculated my days and told myself to wait a little longer. A couple of days later it still hadn't come and so I rather nervously took a pregnancy test. To my utter disbelief, the test came out positive – a strong positive. I stared down at the test, trying to let it all sink in and work out how I was feeling.

Having felt the deep pain of loss, my reaction to being pregnant was mixed and very complex. I felt an overwhelming sense of excitement and terror in equal measure. While I felt joy and some hope that this time might be different, my mind was consumed with anxiety. *Is my body going to do what it should this time? What if this ends the same way it always has? How will I cope if I have another miscarriage?*

Over the next few days, I had the pregnancy confirmed by my fertility specialist. He kindly offered to give me a scan to determine whether everything was as it should be and of course we jumped at the chance. It was so early in the pregnancy that there wasn't much to see on the scan except a small blob and this tiny, beautiful beating heart! It was so amazing to see it right there, beating in front of me, and I was flooded with relief. The doctor told us to come back again two weeks later to check everything had grown as it should. The second scan was even more amazing and showed our little baby had grown, and the heart was still beating strongly.

As we left the clinic, my husband and I finally felt that we could allow ourselves to celebrate and to believe that we would get to hold this baby in our arms. It was a wonderful feeling after having to be so restrained and guarded.

As the days passed between scans and midwife visits, anxious thoughts started to creep back in. What if the heart had stopped beating since we last saw it? I became obsessed about checking for any spotting or bleeding. My work colleagues must have thought I was incontinent because I would go into the toilet every five minutes to check. I would only wear white underwear so that I could easily notice any blood. I also constantly checked my symptoms.

Was I still feeling nausea?

Were my breasts still sore?

If I didn't feel either of these things strongly, I'd become more anxious. It was difficult in these first few months to concentrate on anything else in daily life because my mind was constantly racing with thoughts of whether my baby was still alive. I was fortunate to have a wonderful and supportive sister-in-law who was also a midwife. She was extremely patient with all my questions and concerns and offered to bring her Doppler round on more than one occasion when I was anxious, so that I could hear the heartbeat and be reassured.

As the months went by and I started to feel our baby move, the worry and obsessive toilet visits subsided. I felt more and more at peace that it was all going to be OK.

About halfway through the pregnancy, I finally relaxed and managed to enjoy the wonder of having this miracle growing inside me. I relished every movement I felt, and even the severe pelvic pain I experienced didn't get me down (at least not all the time!).

That October, we finally held our precious baby boy in our arms, and the love, joy and utter relief we felt was overwhelming. I stared in complete wonder at this beautiful gift, aware that the love and gratitude welling

up in my heart were so much deeper because of the
painful journey we'd travelled.

Today I am grateful for

DAY 4

Support – Fear

Fear can dominate our thinking and leave no room for
rational thoughts, so how does one overcome this daily
challenge? I believe the secret lies in the fact that we have
a choice to either focus on what fills us with panic or gaze
upon that which brings us hope.

This doesn't mean we won't experience dread, and it
doesn't mean we won't suffer with anxiety, but it does mean
that when our brain allows us to choose to either think the
best or consider the worst, we decide to hold on to hope with
both hands. When we choose to presume all is OK, rather
than believing everything's gone wrong, we understand it
won't change the final outcome, but it certainly makes the
journey a whole lot more bearable.

So many things used to bring me panic when I was
pregnant. People's comments were often big triggers. Someone
saying something like, 'Wow, you're hardly showing, are
you?' would make me fear that something was wrong, if my
bump was smaller than other people's. Or, 'Are you feeling
the baby move yet, as I did at your gestation?' was another

surefire way to send me hurtling into a world of anxiety. Let me reassure you that every pregnancy is unique, so just because your friend is experiencing XYZ doesn't mean you should be feeling the same. When a wave of panic does hit, just take time to practise your relaxation exercises. Give yourself time to regroup, and then your mind will be in a better place to hear the reassurance you may need to offer it. If you need more assurance that all is well, speak to your midwife.

Today I am grateful for

DAY 5

Journalling your pregnancy

What gestation is your baby today? _____

How big are they? _____

What symptoms are you now feeling?

What do you want to remember about how you are feeling or what you are experiencing?

> When you are harshly criticising yourself,
> as you feel you didn't achieve enough today,
> just remind yourself that purely surviving was enough.
>
> ZOË CLARK-COATES

Today I am grateful for

DAY 6

Support – Expecting to fail

One of the hardest parts of life post-loss is that it can rob you of future excitement. When you have spent so long in fight-

or-flight mode, anything can trigger a reaction, and the way many people respond is to try to protect themselves from disappointment. The way they do this is by trying not to get excited about things (just in case it fails, or doesn't live up to expectations), and of course this limits the life they are living.

Why look forward to Christmas, when someone could easily get sick and the day be ruined?

Why get excited about an evening with friends, when they may cancel at the last minute?

Why plan for a new baby, when you have no assurance you will bring them home?

So many self-protection measures that simply stop you from fully embracing life.

If you can work at stopping catastrophising in your head, it makes a world of difference to how you live your life. Even a few small tweaks to your thought patterns can make life easier for you.

The first task in changing negative thought patterns is to learn what your go-to thought pattern is. Don't judge yourself, just observe. Start to note down your first thoughts when thinking of the future. After a week, look back at your notes, and look for any repeating patterns. Do you naturally think the worst? Is your first response panic? Once you have discovered how your mind works, you can then look at changing your natural responses. Some people need professional help to change thought patterns, but others can do this themselves, just by interrupting the unwanted response with a chosen replacement such as, 'I choose to believe all will be well.'

Today I am grateful for

DAY 7

Journal

What sort of parent do you want to become?

- -

At times you don't need
to seek the light,
it just seems to find you.

- - - - - - - - - - - - ZOË CLARK-COATES - - - - - - - - - - - -

Today I am grateful for

WEEK 14

●●●●●●●●●●●●●●●●●●●●●●●●●●●●●●●●●●●●●●

DAY 1

Support – Fear of others thinking a new baby is a replacement for a child who has died

This is the ultimate fear for so many parents after baby loss, and something I have to reassure people about daily. No baby can replace another; any additional children are beautiful blessings and siblings to those who have run ahead.

So how does one navigate this worry?

I guess one has to accept that we can't control what others think. However much we want those around us to see things the same way we do, we can't demand it. All we can do is share our view and hope others feel the same. I made it clear to everyone close to me that the children we have the honour of raising never replaced those who died. My husband and I felt this was not only important for us, but also for our daughters. That didn't mean people wouldn't occasionally say something that caused upset or express things in ways that caused us offence. But we always trusted that it wasn't anyone's intention to cause us pain, and often it was just their naïvety that made them pick the wrong words.

One real challenge for many is thinking that if their precious baby hadn't died, this current baby wouldn't exist. How does one get their head around that? I don't think you can get your head around it, to be honest, as I don't think it will ever make sense why some people die and some get to live. I think you just have to find peace in the knowledge that while it will never be OK that your baby died, it's OK to celebrate and rejoice that the baby you have with you does get to live. You don't have to be OK with someone dying; you don't have to understand why life has dealt the cards it has.

You just have to find a way of accepting that this is how life has unfolded.

Today I am grateful for

>

DAY 2

Task

Some say grief lessens over time, and for some, maybe it does. My personal opinion is that you just get better equipped at carrying it. Your muscles become stronger over time, so you notice the weight of your pain less often.

How would you describe your grief at the time of loss, and how would you describe it now?

>

Today I am grateful for

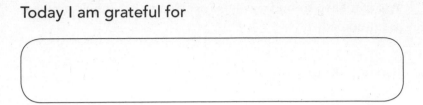

DAY 3

Dr Jessica Farren MA, MBBS, MRCOG, PhD, OBGYN

Why do some people feel exhausted and others energised in pregnancy?

This probably relates to hormones and the individual way every woman responds to them. Just like women have very different experiences of their menstrual cycle – with some women suffering from severe premenstrual syndrome, and others having no symptoms at all – women seem to respond to the rapidly changing hormones in early pregnancy in very different ways. Some feel full of energy and enthusiasm. Others find the hormones can actually make them quite low in mood, which they don't expect, and this can make them feel guilty. Others find their mood and energy levels fluctuate hugely. Some women find these changes persist throughout pregnancy, and others find they plateau, usually sometime in the second trimester.

Women who have sickness and nausea may struggle to eat and drink and may feel exhausted as a result. The important thing is to notice the changes, recognise that that's what your brain and body have decided to do, and be kind to yourself. Don't compare yourself to others – and don't be afraid to be honest about how you're feeling with those close to you, and with your GP.

Why is it common to have aching period-like pain in pregnancy?

By the end of pregnancy, your womb is 500 times its original size! This monumental transformation is bound to come with some 'growing pains'.

It is very common to feel some mild cramps relating to the start of some of this growth in the first few weeks of pregnancy. These may often feel like period pain, which will understandably make most women feel anxious. You may also find you experience some cramping related to constipation, which is a common effect of the pregnancy hormone progesterone. Mild pain, or pain that gets better when you have a rest or change positions, is very unlikely to be anything to worry about.

Pain is also very common in the second trimester – when women are often told they have ligament pain. This represents the time when the womb, having been well supported right inside the pelvis, grows to a size at which it has space to tilt forward and stretch the ligaments that join the sides of the womb to the bones of the pelvis. Sometimes the pain can be quite sharp in nature.

If you experience sudden or severe pain, or if you have any associated bleeding, then you should seek medical advice.

Why do some women bleed in early pregnancy?

Experiencing a few spots of bleeding in early pregnancy is very common, and does not necessarily mean there is a problem. In very early pregnancy, it is the cyst on the ovary (the corpus luteum), from where the egg was released, that produces the hormone progesterone that is responsible for maintaining the pregnancy and stopping you from bleeding. It gets a signal from the very early pregnancy to continue progesterone production – and, as it does, the levels may drop slightly, and you may experience a small amount of bleeding. It is unlikely that this represents the implantation itself – as this is taking place on a microscopic level – but it happens around the time of implantation, hence the name 'implantation bleed'.

Bleeding can also take place as the pregnancy develops, and embeds into the lining of the womb. Sometimes, as it does so, a little bruise beneath the placenta can form (a 'subchorionic haematoma') – and, as this resolves, you may have some brown loss (which represents 'old' rather than fresh blood loss) for a few days or weeks.

Sometimes bleeding can be from the cervix, which responds to the hormones in pregnancy and, as a result, becomes slightly more sensitive (so you are more likely to bleed after sex).

Of course, any bleeding should be investigated. Sadly, it can sometimes represent a miscarriage, or an ectopic pregnancy, especially if it is associated with pain. An ultrasound scan (usually performed as an internal scan in the early stages of pregnancy) is a quick and safe way to make sure things are developing normally, and your GP should be able to help you to arrange to see a specialist for this within a day or two.

Today I am grateful for

DAY 4

Support – Changing relationships

Pregnancy can change so many things about relationships – those with your partner and those with family and friends.

Some people may be happy you are pregnant; others may not be delighted. Sadly (or possibly thankfully) we can't control everything or everyone, so we have to accept that changing circumstances can alter how we relate to one another.

As always, talking is one of the keys to adjusting to new circumstances, so don't be nervous about opening up conversations with those closest to you.

When you discover you are pregnant, you can instantly feel different. Your priorities and motivations change and, while it feels like the most natural thing in the world for you, it can be surprisingly hard for those around you. I have heard some people say, 'I felt like I lost my best friend overnight, as suddenly she could only focus on the baby.' I raise this subject to encourage you to look at things from every angle, as pregnancy can be hard on those around us. I always encourage people to look outside of their life as much as possible, not only to ensure friendships and relationships are protected, but also to ensure your world doesn't become too insular.

While I was pregnant, I made sure I texted my friends regularly, asking about their lives, to ensure they still felt I cared about what was going on for them – as I did care! I made sure I sent birthday cards etc. and I made notes about things they said, so I would remember to ask them about what was going on in their lives, even while I was preoccupied with being pregnant. In my experience good relationships take work, and any time you can invest will pay you dividends later.

Today I am grateful for

DAY 5

Journalling your pregnancy

What gestation is your baby today? _____

How big are they? _____

What symptoms are you now feeling?

What do you want to remember about how you are feeling
or what you are experiencing?

. . . .

The pain may feel too big for you to carry,
but that is why you have people in your corner.
They may not be able to carry your loss,
but they can help carry you.

. . . . ZOË CLARK-COATES . . . .

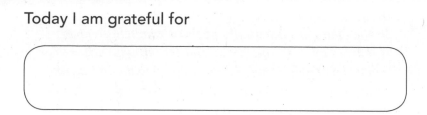

Today I am grateful for

DAY 6

Support – Judgement

Why, oh why do we all fear being judged by others?

Perhaps you are worried that people may think you are grieving for too long? Maybe you are concerned that friends are thinking you aren't enjoying your pregnancy as much as you should be?

What I have learnt is this: we cannot control what anyone else thinks. By allowing that worry to fester, we are inadvertently giving away our power to others. We are literally allowing fear to change the way we live. I can't tell you that no one is judging you, as sadly this is part of human nature – everyone judges those around them. Yes, some do it more harshly than others, but everyone does it to some extent. However, we can all choose how we react to it.

We can decide not to inhabit that place of worry, and we can say, 'Whatever others think, I am going to live in a way I am comfortable with.' When we boldly step out of the box of conformity and live bravely, I promise you life becomes more manageable, as you can be genuinely authentic in everything you do.

One of my favourite quotes about judgement is this, from Theodore Roosevelt:

> *It is not the critic who counts; not the man who points out how the strong man stumbles, or where the doer of*

deeds could have done them better. The credit belongs to the man who is actually in the arena, whose face is marred by dust and sweat and blood; who strives valiantly; who errs, who comes short again and again, because there is no effort without error and shortcoming; but who does actually strive to do the deeds; who knows great enthusiasms, the great devotions; who spends himself in a worthy cause; who at the best knows in the end the triumph of high achievement, and who at the worst, if he fails, at least fails while daring greatly, so that his place shall never be with those cold and timid souls who neither know victory nor defeat.

Today I am grateful for

DAY 7

Journal

What do you cherish most about your life?

If you could create your perfect day out, what would it be?

The world may try to rush you to heal,
rush you to feel, rush you to move on.
Let me reassure you of this.

You can stand still or you can walk slow.
You can swim against the current,
or just move with the waves.

You, my friend, can take
all the time you need.

ZOË CLARK-COATES

Today I am grateful for

WEEK 15

· ·

DAY 1

Support – I remember

I remember days when I felt so overwhelmed, and I would sit on my bathroom floor having no clue how I would get through a whole pregnancy feeling so scared. That is the issue with worry – it consumes us, and it can make us feel almost hopeless.

So how did I get through it? By forcing myself to not look so far in advance.

I constantly reminded myself that I didn't have to get through nine months feeling like that, as each day I felt different things. Some days I was filled with hope and positivity, while other days felt scary and challenging.

The skills I learnt in pregnancy – staying present, holding on to hope, banishing anxiety – all then helped me parent better when the girls arrived in my arms, so nothing you learn now will be wasted. Just take it a day at a time. You don't need to find the strength to get through tomorrow; you only need to make it through this day. Tomorrow you will wake with the strength you need for the next 24 hours.

Today I am grateful for

DAY 2

Task

I want you to put a relaxing piece of music on and lie down. Now I want you to imagine you have delivered your baby and you are now sitting looking at them in your arms. Sit with this image in your mind. Feel it. Believe it. This is your end goal and having a clear mental image of it in your mind can help you through hard times.

(The music I used for this visualisation exercise randomly came on the radio in the recovery room when I was holding my daughter immediately following her birth. I can't even begin to tell you what a special moment that was!)

Today I am grateful for

DAY 3

Jill's Story

I was blessed to give birth to our daughter. She was our first child, and even though I didn't have a great pregnancy, she was born a good weight and healthy.

Some years later we decided to try for another child, but we sadly lost the baby through a ruptured ectopic pregnancy, and I was rushed into hospital for a lifesaving operation. A year later we lost another baby through early miscarriage. Our lives had been turned upside down, and we felt broken. Our hearts were in a million pieces.

Then I fell pregnant with our fourth baby; as I stared at the lines on the pregnancy test, my heart skipped a beat (well, to be honest, it skipped several beats). In that moment I was so overwhelmed with happiness, joy, hopes and dreams, because after many years of trying for another baby and after many negative pregnancy tests, there they were – the two lines that I was longing to see. But then the fear gripped me. Would we lose this baby as well?

Could my heart take another loss? So many questions were racing around my head.

As with all the other pregnancies, we told people as soon as we found out that we were expecting. This was mostly met with joy and congratulations, but a few people said we shouldn't announce it so early, you know . . . just in case it happened again. That way we wouldn't have to deal with telling people we lost another baby. I know they meant well, but to us, that was saying that our baby wasn't worth celebrating and also that we shouldn't talk about the babies we lost. Perhaps it was for their benefit, so they didn't have to see us sad and grieving, or for our benefit, so we didn't have to hear the words, 'Oh no, not again.'

There were so many emotions to deal with . . .

I remember being obsessed with going to the toilets just to check to see if there was any sign of miscarriage. Every time we were out, I would be mentally checking where all the toilets were so I could go and check just to make sure it wasn't happening again. Every twinge or pain sent me into a spin . . . and I would feel crippled with fear and panic.

Every scan I had (and there were many) was a reminder of the day we heard those heart-wrenching words, *'I'm so sorry, there is no heartbeat and your baby has died.'*

Every time I lay on the couch in the ultrasound room, I would unconsciously hold my breath until I heard my baby's heart beating. The relief was overwhelming that we'd made it through another week and my baby was still alive and growing.

I would long for the nine months to rush by so I could hold my baby in my arms, something that I so desperately wanted to do with the babies I lost.

Pregnancy should be a time of joy and anticipation, but for me, it was filled with worry, fear, 'what ifs' and lots of tears! I felt the joy of expecting another baby was stolen from me and I was hanging on with gritted teeth, wishing the time away. My every waking moment was spent thinking and praying that our baby would survive another day.

There were times I would feel happy and was so thankful that we were having another baby, but this was always overshadowed by fear and anxiety.

It wasn't until much later in the pregnancy that I began to relax and not feel so worried. I can remember feeling the first proper kick and being so happy, but I also felt sad that I didn't get a chance to feel that before with the babies we had lost.

During the whole pregnancy, I didn't really talk about my fears and worries to anyone. I thought that some people would think I was silly; I guess I thought no one else would understand how I was feeling. I realise now that not talking about my feelings only made it worse. I would make up all sorts of scenarios in my head which only led to me feeling more anxious.

My time then came and I gave birth to a healthy boy.

Eighteen months later I was pregnant with our fifth baby. I thought this time I would be OK, and all the feelings and worries I experienced with my last pregnancy wouldn't happen this time. How wrong could I be! If anything, my anxieties were worse than before. I spent most days crying and totally consumed with guilt that I felt this way.

It was so easy to get caught up in my own grief, pain, fear and worry that I forgot about how my family were feeling. Because I didn't open up and show them how I really was, they felt they couldn't express how they were feeling either.

I would put on a brave face, especially in front of our daughter. I wanted to protect her, so she didn't have to feel what I felt. I tried to keep this to myself, but on one visit to the midwife, I totally broke down and couldn't get my words out. I had bottled everything up for so long that I just couldn't cope anymore. That particular visit to the health visitor ended up with me being diagnosed with prenatal depression. Don't get me wrong, I desperately wanted this baby and was happy I was pregnant, but I couldn't shake this awful fear that was eating me up.

It was then that I had to be honest with myself and those close to me. I wasn't some kind of superwoman who could just soldier on and not face up to my real feelings. It was time for me to be real, and to realise that everything I was feeling was quite normal. The emotional rollercoaster I was on was all part of my journey in this particular season of my life.

I realised the way for me to move forward and find joy amid the fear, anxiety and pain was to talk, no matter how daft I felt or how worried that I would make people feel awkward.

I then gave birth to another son. I had completed my family. I will never forget those years filled with both joy and tears.

Today I am grateful for

DAY 4

Support – Delaying peace

It is super-common to delay peace or happiness by thinking, 'I'll be happy when . . .'

In a pregnancy following a baby loss, we may put off allowing ourselves to feel certain things until we get to a specified gestation or even to the birth. Most people find the goalposts steadily get moved further and further back. 'I will be happy following my 20-week scan' suddenly changes to 'I will be happy at 37 weeks of pregnancy', and that then changes to 'I will be happy once they are born', and before you know it that changes to 'I will be happy when they are three months old'.

Your fear is robbing you of so many happy moments in the present.

Don't get me wrong, I know this is easy to say and hard to do in practice, but I beg you to allow yourself to celebrate every little milestone.

- Enjoy every kick, every movement – you, yes YOU, deserve to be happy RIGHT now.
- So relax (as much as possible).
- Don't let fear rob you of the gift of the present moment.
- The gift that right now all is OK.
- Right now, you are pregnant.
- Right now, you have survived some serious crap, and are still standing.
- Right now – it's OK to be happy, and it is OK to embrace peace.

Today I am grateful for

DAY 5

Journalling your pregnancy

What gestation is your baby today? _____

How big are they? _____

What symptoms are you now feeling?

What do you want to remember about how you are feeling
or what you are experiencing?

The struggle is real, but you are worth every worry,
every sleepless night, and every tormented day.

ZOË CLARK-COATES

Today I am grateful for

DAY 6

Support – Answering the question, 'Is this your first child?'

Responding to this question can throw people into a whirlwind
of panic. You don't want to ever deny a child who has died,

but do you want to get into such an in-depth conversation with a random stranger? Let me assure you there is no right or wrong way to navigate this. You, and only you, determine what you feel comfortable sharing and revealing.

When people ask this question, what I tend to assume they are asking is, 'Do you have other children you are raising?' rather than, 'Is this the first time your womb has carried a child?' So I never felt like I was lying if I said, 'Yes.' However, I would mostly say, 'I have children in heaven already.'

This meant I spent a lot of time making sure other people were OK, as people would then worry that they had asked an inappropriate question, and I felt that rubbish need to make them feel OK about me being potentially upset. But it was an answer I felt comfortable giving and the more I said it, the better I became at handling any reaction I was met with.

Having pre-set answers can help navigate these complex situations. When you know you can handle any polite or not-so-polite question, you feel more confident in being out in the world.

So I encourage you to spend time thinking what your answers will be, and then practise them when it's just you sitting in front of a mirror. Get comfortable with the words, so they roll off your tongue without panic engulfing you.

I know another big concern for many who have lost a child through miscarriage is that society will make them feel silly for considering that a baby lost at an early gestation is a baby. They fear that because, medically, these little ones aren't recognised as children, a parent will be seen as exaggerating the loss or making it seem more than it is. Let me reassure you that, whatever stage you lost your baby, you lost your child. It doesn't matter what anyone else thinks or believes; the only thing that matters is what you and your partner feel. So please try to let this fear go if you are carrying it.

Today I am grateful for

[ ]

DAY 7

Journal

What traditions would you like to offer to your children?

[ ]

· ·

To the one who feels it is just too much to carry,
I promise you have the strength.

· · · · · · · · · · · ZOË CLARK-COATES · · · · · · · · · · ·

Today I am grateful for

[ ]

WEEK 16

. . . .

DAY 1

Support – How to handle the judgement from those around you who simply don't understand loss and the fear of trying for more babies

It never fails to amaze me the things people feel in a position to judge. It would never even occur to me to judge or comment on someone's choices to have or not have children, but many people do feel they can comment. I quite regularly hear people saying, 'I just can't believe they keep putting themselves through more losses.' It takes everything in my power to keep my mouth shut. They are not 'putting themselves through loss'; they are trying to grow their family and have a precious child.

So how should one handle any judgement or lack of sympathy about loss or pregnancy?

- Firstly, you have to try (and this is hard) not to care about anyone else's opinion. These judgemental views hold no power over you unless you give them space and allow them to influence your thinking. If they aren't helpful or a blessing to you, disregard them as unimportant.
- Secondly, I have sadly found that the path of pregnancy after baby loss is pretty hard to comprehend unless you have walked down it. Even if you explained your experience and feelings until the end of time, that would only give others a snippet of insight into it. So pick your battles wisely, and only spend time explaining to people who you genuinely care about.

I hope that my words within these pages show you there is someone out there who gets what you feel.

Today I am grateful for

DAY 2

Task

Why should you be proud of yourself? Write to yourself saying all the things you would say to a friend who was walking a similar path to you.

Dear me

Today I am grateful for

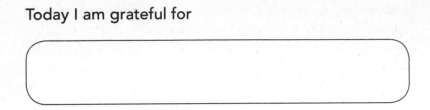

DAY 3

Registered Dietician Nichola Ludlam-Raine BSc (Hons), PG Dip, MSc

We covered food advice earlier in the book, but now would be a good time to recap. What foods should one eat to keep a baby healthy in the womb?

A healthy diet is important at any time. However, it is vital for mums-to-be as demands on the body are increased during pregnancy. Eating a balanced diet will help your baby to grow and develop, and you'll be less likely to suffer from complications. You don't need to eat a special diet, but you do need to pay attention to what you're eating, ensuring that you eat a variety of different foods to obtain all the nutrients that you and your baby need.

A healthy and balanced diet consists of eating plenty of fruit and vegetables for vitamins, minerals and fibre, which will help to keep you healthy and prevent constipation. Ideally we should be eating between five and nine portions of fruit and vegetables a day, with a portion being around a handful or 80g; for example, an apple, a small bowl of salad or three tablespoons of peas. Aim to fill around a third of your meal plate with vegetables or salad and if you're hungry between meals have a piece of fruit; to jazz it up, you could have a banana with nut butter or an apple with cheese.

Protein, which includes meat, fish, eggs, beans, pulses, milk, cheese and yoghurt, should take up another third of your plate or bowl, as our bodies and babies need protein daily to grow and also repair. Aim to eat two portions of fish a week, one of which is oily, e.g. salmon, mackerel or sardines (avoid shark, marlin and swordfish, though, because of mercury levels in larger fish). Make sure that all of your foods are cooked thoroughly to prevent food poisoning and choose leaner cuts of meat where possible, avoiding liver as it contains too much vitamin A, which can be harmful in pregnancy. If you really don't feel like eating, due to morning sickness for example, then a glass of milk is ideal as it will provide you with calcium, protein and slow-release energy, as well as keeping you hydrated.

Wholegrain or slow-release starchy carbohydrates such as sweet potato, oats, wholemeal pasta, basmati rice or granary bread provide your body with B vitamins, energy and fibre. Aim to fill another third of your plate with these to keep you fuelled for the entire day.

Keeping hydrated is also important as it will help to keep your digestive system moving and gut healthy. Aim for your urine to be a pale straw colour!

Focus on what you should be eating more of, and you'll naturally eat less of the foods high in sugar and fat and low in nutrients, such as cake and biscuits; these can, however, be enjoyed in moderation (especially with friends over coffee!).

What can you eat to reduce acid and reflux?

Foods commonly linked with reflux include fried foods, spicy dishes (such as curries), excessive amounts of caffeine (found in tea, coffee, colas and energy drinks) and alcohol. During pregnancy, alcohol should be strictly avoided, and caffeine should be limited to no more than 200mg a day (the equivalent of two cups of tea or instant coffee a day). Try to eat little and often, as opposed to large meals, and remember

to *chew your food well. You may also want to avoid eating
your meal within two hours of bedtime, so that digestion
doesn't interfere with your sleep.*

What foods can you eat to keep your blood sugars stable?

*Make sure the carbohydrates that you eat are low glycaemic
index (GI), meaning the energy/glucose is released relatively
slowly. Low GI carbs include: pasta, sweet potatoes, rye or
granary bread, oats, muesli, pulses, lentils or basmati rice.
Fill one quarter to one third of your plate with starchy carbs,
depending on how active you are (a fist-sized serving is ample,
though, for most people), along with a source of protein and
vegetables to lower the GI even further.*

What foods can I eat to help with nausea?

*Eating little and often may help with nausea, so too will
dry foods such as oatcakes or rice cakes. Anecdotal research
also suggests that ginger may help to alleviate symptoms. If
the smell of hot food makes you feel sick, have cold foods
instead, such as sandwiches or cereal.*

What foods can I eat to increase my energy levels?

*Regular meals are essential for sustaining energy levels and
sitting down to eat as a family will help to teach good table
manners, as well as encouraging children to try new foods.*

*The simplest way to create a balanced plate is to divide
it into thirds as mentioned above, and fill one third with
vegetables or salad, one third with wholegrains or slow-release
carbohydrates such as sweet potato or basmati rice and one
third with lean protein such as chicken, eggs, tuna or a bean
burger. To finish, you can add a small number of healthy fats
in the form of olive oil, avocado, seeds or feta cheese for taste.*

What food can I eat to help me sleep better?

Avoid having a large meal or bedtime snack as you may feel uncomfortably full getting to sleep and this could even lead to heartburn, which may make sleep worse. Have your evening meal ideally at least two to three hours before bed and keep it to one dinner plate size!

A glass of milk may aid sleep as it provides protein, carbohydrates and calcium, which helps the brain to convert tryptophan into the sleep-inducing substance serotonin.

The best way of ensuring optimal melatonin production (which also helps you to sleep) is to make your bedroom as dark as possible – light suppresses the production of it.

What food can I eat after having my baby to increase my milk supply?

There's limited evidence that certain foods help to boost milk supply; the best thing to do is to eat a healthy and balanced diet with a sufficient amount of calories (honouring your hunger), stay hydrated and feed on demand.

Today I am grateful for

DAY 4

Support – Excitement and fear

People often ask me why they get struck by panic even when they are doing something they love, and that is a great question. Excitement and fear can bring about the same cortisol swell, so when we get that sense of excitement in our stomachs, our brains can respond in a similar way as they do when we feel nervous, and our fight-or-flight response can kick in and make us want to run for the hills. That's how you can go from looking forward to a fun event one moment, to utter panic about it in the blink of an eye.

You can learn to switch off or reduce this response, but it takes time and effort. I think just understanding why it happens can make people feel less confused when they experience it.

Sadly, most people don't ever address the core reasons why this happens. This can mean that, over time, they limit their activities and avoid anything that makes them either excited or nervous. This avoidance tactic shrinks their world and robs them of an abundance of life opportunities.

If you experience this sensation please can I encourage you to address it, perhaps with professional help. In the meantime, I would suggest you practise mindfulness and relaxation techniques to help you cope with any feelings of panic that spontaneously surface. You need to try to calm and soothe your fight-or-flight response and regulate your breathing.

Today I am grateful for

DAY 5

Journalling your pregnancy

What gestation is your baby today? _____

How big are they? _____

What symptoms are you now feeling?

What do you want to remember about how you are feeling or what you are experiencing?

. . . .

Focusing on gratitude really
helped me navigate pregnancy.

When I could feel myself spiralling
into panic I would calmly repeat
to myself over and over again,
'I am so thankful you are here',
while stroking my stomach.

It is amazing how feeling thankful can
silence that voice of fear.

. . . . ZOË CLARK-COATES . . . .

Today I am grateful for

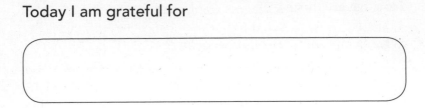

DAY 6

Support – Fear of labour and delivery

Just because you dearly want to raise a baby doesn't mean you are expected to be fearless around everything to do with creating and delivering a baby. Often people say to me, 'How can I be scared of something I have been longing to do?' I always explain that they have every right to be anxious, and they are as justified as anyone else to be nervous or fearful. I also hear from many people who are so frightened about the delivery of their child it prevents them from being able to enjoy their pregnancy, as the fear is constantly hovering overhead.

First, let's look at what you are nervous of.

If you have previously delivered a baby who didn't live, this will of course have dramatically impacted your views and expectations around subsequent births. I would suggest talking as much as possible about all previous birth experiences and any and all emotions that surrounded them, either to a friend or to a professional counsellor.

- Try to determine where your fear lies.
- Are you nervous about the physical pain?
- Are you scared of feeling out of control?
- Are you worried about going into hospital?
- Are you afraid of your baby being poorly or not surviving?

- Once you identify the specific issues that are making you anxious, you can chat about them, and hopefully have those around you reassure you.
- Often the things we fear and keep internalised grow bigger and bigger. When you verbalise them, you may find they lose some of their power.

Today I am grateful for

DAY 7

Journal

What character traits would you like your children to have and why?

This is when I would normally remind you
that whatever this week throws at you,
you can handle it.

But instead, I will whisper it's OK to have
moments when you feel you can't cope.

It is fine to not know how you will survive
the next 24 hours.

It is understandable that you want to just lie
on the floor screaming that life isn't fair.

You may not feel you have the strength to
continue, my friend, but I
promise that you do.

ZOË CLARK-COATES

Today I am grateful for

WEEK 17

● ●

DAY 1

Support – Fearing a lack of attachment to the baby

What stops you from allowing yourself to fully feel an attachment can of course be fear. Fear of pain, fear of grief, fear of loss. But trying not to have an attachment to a baby doesn't actually protect people from the pain of loss. If you lose a baby you still grieve, you still break, you still mourn whether you felt you had an attachment or not. You may try to kid yourself that it wouldn't hurt as much if you were to stay detached, but that isn't the truth. If you lose something that you love, you grieve.

So is self-protection always wrong?

Of course not; to some degree self-protection is essential. If we want to get something out of the oven, we protect our hands with oven gloves. We don't just say, 'I'm starving, and my dinner is ready in the oven, but as I am too scared I will get burnt, I am just going to leave it in there.' We put oven gloves on and safely get the food out and put it on our plates. Likewise, there are vital things that we can do to help protect ourselves and our babies . . . a healthy lifestyle, eating right, not drinking alcohol or smoking, etc. We can also protect ourselves emotionally by not jumping too far ahead, as this helps us stay in the present and not worry (as much) about tomorrow.

So isn't stopping oneself bonding just essential self-protection?

Self-protection may be the reason we try to detach from our growing baby, but it doesn't help us during a pregnancy after loss. Detachment doesn't stop any pain, it just brings guilt and conflict to our hearts and minds. Nature determines that we love and cherish our offspring, and if we fight these natural urges, we are just creating mental conflict for ourselves and, potentially, further issues down the line.

Sometimes we need to take the risk of putting all our eggs in one basket. We have to trust everything will work out and, if the basket breaks, we trust that we have the strength to survive and move forward. At times this means going against what society and those around us tell us. 'Don't get excited until after your 12-week scan.' 'Don't bond until you know all is well.' I believe this is actually unhelpful advice as it's asking you to go against how your natural emotional response was created to react. So be led by your heart and trust me when I tell you it is OK to love your baby from the second you see those two pink lines on a pregnancy test.

Today I am grateful for

DAY 2

Task

Fill this box with words that describe how you are feeling right now. Write the words in different sizes, with the emotions you feel strongest in the largest letters.

Today I am grateful for

DAY 3

Gemma's Story

It is such a cliché but going for my scan post-baby loss was a rollercoaster of emotions. This was my fourth pregnancy, but I only had one living child.

For so long, I had wanted and needed another baby in my life. A baby for me, and a sibling for my son. I don't consider myself a religious person, but I found it was all I prayed for.

When I finally discovered I was pregnant again, I knew this would be my last pregnancy, my last ever chance. I promised myself that I would enjoy every single moment, every milestone I managed to reach; I promised to cherish every part of the pregnancy, good and bad.

Instead, I found myself constantly at war with my emotions. When it wasn't a battle between joy and fear, it was guilt. Guilt that I wasn't happy enough, that I was focusing too much on past grief and not enough on my current happiness; I wasn't appreciating the miracle of my prayers being answered. Guilt when I was happy, like somehow that meant I had forgotten or replaced my lost babies.

Every time I felt any twinge or unusual sensation, I worried something was going wrong. When I didn't feel symptoms, I convinced myself there was a problem.

I couldn't bear the thought of waiting weeks for my 12-week scan, not knowing if my worst fears were happening all over again, so I booked myself in for an early private scan.

Sitting in the waiting room, I tried to prepare myself for 'the look' and the phrase 'I'm so sorry'. I'd heard it before and felt sure I was about to hear it again. But it didn't come; there was a heartbeat, and a little wriggly bean, shaped like a bunny rabbit!

Somewhere along the way of my baby journey, I lost the ability to believe in my body and what it could achieve. I needed something physical to hold on to. For me, it was the scans. With each one, I grew in confidence that everything was going to be OK and that I could enjoy this pregnancy.

Throughout the rest of the pregnancy, I had several complications, which brought all the fear and anxiety right back to the surface.

But ultimately, we survived, together.

I held on to the joy and the milestones as tightly as I could, until the day I got to bring my baby home.

Home to his bunny-rabbit-themed nursery and excited big brother.

Today I am grateful for

DAY 4

Support – Fear of loss when the baby is born

I remember expecting that the fear would just vanish when my baby was born safely. I had no idea that my worry would transfer to fear over my child then staying alive. This is why I encourage everyone to deal with their anxiety during pregnancy, as it can genuinely rob you of peace when your baby is born, and throughout their childhood. Practise stopping terror in its tracks by starving the fear. Refuse to enter into the dialogue of torment, which will have you running through a million disaster possibilities in your mind.

If your parents or people who raised you (or influenced you) were worriers, it's highly likely that you have learnt from their example. You may be an expert at spinning an entirely innocent situation into a danger-filled catastrophe in your imagination. I have found that those who taught us how to worry are usually able to intensify our fear like no one else. You may innocently share something with them and, before you can count to 10, they have made you spiral into a whole new level of panic. This is because they hold keys to your doors of fear.

If this sounds familiar, I encourage you to be careful what you choose to share with this person. Let me give you an example of this. My mum is prone to panic when it comes to issues around finance. If I ever shared with her any money worries, she would freak out, and this then made me panic way more. I found I was then carrying my anxiety, plus hers, and my fear was now a hundred times bigger than it was before our discussion. I learnt to handle this by not talking about money issues with my mum. This not only helped me but it also, in turn, helped her, as it gave her one less thing to be concerned about. When it comes to talking about hopes and dreams, however, my mum would be one of the first people I would turn to; she would never trigger me to panic over future plans, she would just help me to figure a way forward. So consider carefully what to share with different people in your life; it is perfectly OK to have a few off-limits subjects, even with those closest to you.

Today I am grateful for

DAY 5

Journalling your pregnancy

What gestation is your baby today? _____

How big are they? _____

What symptoms are you now feeling?

What do you want to remember about how you are feeling or what you are experiencing?

I lost my heart to you, little one,
forever, for always it's yours.

ZOË CLARK-COATES

Today I am grateful for

DAY 6

Support – Purchasing baby items

I am often asked when it is 'safe' to begin buying clothes and other items for the new baby. My answer is always this: 'When you want to and feel ready.'

No one should tell you it is too soon or too late to think about preparing for your baby's arrival; the only important thing is you feel ready and want to do it.

I bought baby clothes from the moment I had my first scan. For me, preparing for my little one's arrival was exciting, and I didn't want to delay it. I did, however, wait until the final trimester to purchase more significant items like a pram and a cot. This hesitation was not, as you might think, in case my baby died, but because I didn't want to have a house full of equipment taking up space long before I was ready to use it. So I advise you to buy things when you want to. The purchasing of new baby items can be joy-filled moments. They are times to cherish, to get excited about and to help you look positively to the future, so don't let anyone rob you of them (including yourself!).

Today I am grateful for

DAY 7

Journal

What scares you most in life, outside of this pregnancy? Explain why.

Do you have any irrational fears surrounding this pregnancy?
If yes, how do you feel you can overcome them?

My fear is

and I can overcome it by

* *

Your fear will tell you to prepare for a disaster,
but it is simply not possible to
prepare for heartbreak.

Instead one should focus on a
hope-filled future, and in turn you will be
rewarded with peace.

* * * * * * * * * * * ZOË CLARK-COATES * * * * * * * * * * * *

Today I am grateful for

WEEK 18

● ●

DAY 1

Support – When people don't show up for you

When people fail to show up for us or when they're unable to offer adequate understanding, it can be so hard. Often people assume that a new pregnancy following a loss means a new, entirely positive chapter has been opened. As such, they may not want to discuss a previous loss or the fears that surround pregnancy. This can be incredibly difficult for the expecting parent who is still processing and grieving a baby loss.

A new pregnancy may be the start of a new life growing within, but the one or ones who have died are as much part of this chapter as they were in the last. Additionally, the fears a person is trying to process and deal with need to be discussed and managed to avoid them feeling overwhelmed and consumed.

So how do we address this with those we love? How do we help them to help us?

Firstly, I would ask you to ask yourself one big question. Do people know that you need help or support? Have you communicated your need to them openly? Sometimes we spend so much time and effort trying to look OK that those around us assume we have it all together or don't need help. If you're very good at putting on a brave face, it might not occur to others that you need assistance.

If you are treading water right now, let people know. Speak up and be honest about your struggles – please don't drown when you are surrounded by lifeguards who can throw you a lifebuoy.

*So you have plucked up the courage to speak out –
what next?*

I would advise that you create a circle of support around
yourself. A good exercise is to write a list of all the friends or
family members you would naturally choose to share your
anxieties with.

- Out of those people, who do you feel offers the best
  listening ear?
- Who provides the best practical advice?
- Who helps you escape reality and makes you feel joy and
  happiness?
- Who understands grief and can make you feel less alone
  on this journey through mourning?

This information should help you decide who to share
what with. Remember – you don't need to tell everything to
everyone. Be aware that some people don't have the ability
to offer emotional empathy, and they may be incapable of
offering the support you may need. This doesn't make them
bad friends; it just means you need to be selective in what
you share with them.

Remember that if someone you know is grieving, they
may not be in a position to support you well, but they could
possibly sit and cry with you which can also be a gift.

I am often asked if it's best to share in a group setting with
friends or on a one-to-one basis. Generally, I advise sharing
one to one. My reason is that you may find you need to share
the same story, or worry, over and over to help you process
your feelings. By talking with people individually you can say
the same things without the concern of repeating yourself to
them.

So how honest should we be?

Be as real and honest as possible with those you love and
trust. If you find it difficult to speak out loud, try writing

your feelings down in an email or letter. People aren't mind readers, and if you want them to truly understand, you need to ensure they are fully aware of how you are feeling.

Sadly, grief can change the dynamics of any relationship, and this can be hard to witness and experience. If your friendships change and aren't beneficial to you or them anymore, it's OK to move on and say maybe that friendship was just for a season and not for life. By letting go of outdated friendships, you allow that space to be filled with a new friend who can journey life with you.

When you are inviting people to support you through hard times, you do need to accept that people will mess up . . . this is just a sad part of life. If you can manage your expectations and be ready to forgive when those around you fail, it is easier to retain quality friendships when going through challenges. Don't get me wrong, I'm not saying this will be simple; when you are feeling such pain and anxiety it can be hard to act rationally and it's easy to lose patience with people we think should know better. But if we can show grace to those we love, it can help in the long term.

Today I am grateful for

DAY 2

Task

Many of us defer tasks that fail to bring us joy, but this can increase anxiety levels. Have you been putting off doing things that relate to your pregnancy, or to general life? Have you needed to make certain calls? Write certain letters? Tackle certain jobs? Book certain appointments? Every time you think about the thing you have delayed, you may find you get a wave of panic, and flutters of anxiety, so call a halt to it by just facing it and doing the task this week. In future it is a great practice to do the most stressful things first thing each morning, as then they are out of the way, and you can focus on other things throughout the day without anxiety hovering over you.

What are you prone to putting off? Write a list and then try to do those things first in the future.

_____

_____

_____

_____

_____

_____

_____

Today I am grateful for

DAY 3

Dr Jacque Gerrard MBE, Midwife Consultant and
former Director for England at the Royal College
of Midwives

**Do midwives mind being asked lots of questions and
dealing with your worries?**

*Midwives absolutely love women asking them questions
about their pregnancy and care. It is why we choose
midwifery as a profession. We encourage all women to ask
as many questions as needed to ensure the mother and baby
are well, physically and emotionally, with the healthiest of
outcomes. We want the woman to enjoy her pregnancy as it
is a very special time.*

Are you able to request to change midwives?

*Yes. If you do not have a positive relationship with your
midwife, then contact the head of midwifery to share your
concerns and a change of midwife can be arranged.*

Today I am grateful for

DAY 4

Support – Going on trips while pregnant

For some, getting away from it all is vital to their sanity, while for others, home is where they feel safe and secure and going away feels too much to handle. There is no right or wrong, and only you know what you are comfortable doing.

When people need a break, but want to stay near to their hospital or doctors, I encourage them to just book a hotel near home. You don't have to go on a long flight or travel hours in the car to feel like you are going on holiday. My husband and I have stayed in hotels just an hour away from our house, and it's felt like we're in a different country, thanks to the change of scenery.

Is travelling overseas advisable?

This comes down to how well you are physically and mentally, but if you feel up to it and your medical team say it's OK, go and enjoy your trip. I had a few key requirements when I travelled to places when pregnant; these were:

- A good hospital nearby that I knew cared for babies at the gestation I was (some hospitals only look after babies post 30 weeks, for instance, while others have units for babies from 23 weeks).
- I wanted to be able to easily communicate with any medical teams should I require their care, so I needed to know they spoke my language, or I spoke theirs.
- Finally, I wanted to be able to drive back from wherever we went if I needed to come home quickly – I didn't want to have to board a flight (so this ruled out travelling to the States when I was pregnant).

As long as I could arrange all of these things, I felt OK going away. I have to admit I was happiest when I was at home, however, as I liked knowing the people I trusted medically were all nearby.

So many people used to say to me, 'Enjoy this time, go travel, it's your final time of being alone as a couple.' I think when you have waited so long to become parents, comments like this fall on deaf ears, but there is some truth in it.

Try to appreciate any periods of time you have to talk and bond as a couple before the baby arrives. Embrace opportunities to do activities and learn new things together. The greatest gift you can give to any child is security and a happy home, so never neglect your relationship with your partner.

Today I am grateful for

DAY 5

Journalling your pregnancy

What gestation is your baby today? _____

How big are they? _____

What symptoms are you now feeling?

What do you want to remember about how you are feeling or what you are experiencing?

Some may disappoint you,
but others, they will amaze you.

ZOË CLARK-COATES

Today I am grateful for

DAY 6

Support – Keeping your pregnancy a secret to protect yourself emotionally

Some people find it is helpful to tell people the moment they discover they are pregnant; others find it's more beneficial to keep their pregnancy private. There is no right or wrong way to handle this; it's about what you feel best doing. My only advice is this: if you want other people to feel invested in your pregnancy, they need to know you are pregnant.

I often have people tell me they are upset that their friends weren't overly excited about the birth of their baby. When I ask more questions, it often emerges that they kept the pregnancy private until the baby's birth and now their friends feel rejection that they weren't informed before that point. Their friends also then don't feel bonded to their newborn. This is just something to bear in mind and weigh up. Friends are friends for a reason; we should be able to trust them and include them in our lives even if we share limited information with them.

I love hearing about my friends' pregnancy news. I love looking at their scan pictures, and I adore watching them prepare to become parents, so I know many others will feel the same. Let your friends in, and let them form an attachment with your precious baby.

Today I am grateful for

DAY 7

Journal

If you could set out three intentions for the next three years, what would they be? For example, visiting somewhere, becoming something, or learning a new skill.

1 _____

2 _____

3 _____

• •

Fears can become coal
in a furnace of hope.

• • • • • • • • • • • • ZOË CLARK-COATES • • • • • • • • • • • •

Today I am grateful for

WEEK 19

● ●

DAY 1

Support – Having a health advocate

Having someone who can advocate for you and your needs can be essential for so many people at this time. It's often hard to speak up for oneself, and if you are scared or anxious your brain can feel like mush. This can make it hard even to remember what you want to ask. This is when a family member or friend can become your valuable health advocate.

So what does a health advocate do? Ideally, they accompany you on visits to the doctor, midwife and hospital. It may be helpful if you create a list of questions before the appointment to ensure you get the answers you need. If you are unable to ask the questions, your advocate is there to do so, and this ensures the time you spend with your doctor or midwife etc. is beneficial to you, as well as to the baby.

If your health advocate can accompany you to medical appointments, they can speak up for you if they feel something needs to be said, and they can also ensure that any answer you have been given satisfies you. If you feel confused or uncertain, your advocate can ask the doctor or midwife, 'Can you explain that again, so we both understand?'

This is an important role, so it is vital that you only pick someone you can wholeheartedly trust to be your health advocate. You need someone who won't let you down. Some people make their partners their health advocate, while for others it is better to have an independent third party. If you think you would benefit from having a health advocate on this pregnancy journey, consider all your family and friends who may be up for the task. Carefully consider all the skills they have, and, just as importantly, consider whether their lives would allow them to show up for the next nine months. Make sure you ask them if they have the capacity – emotionally as well as time-wise – to take on this valuable role in your pregnancy.

Today I am grateful for

DAY 2

Task

Create a jar, and each day add in a note stating two things you love about being pregnant. It's OK to repeat things. This jar of notes will become a beautiful keepsake when you have your baby in your arms.

Today I am grateful for

Claire's Story

I'm afraid I am going to use an awful cliché . . . I never thought miscarriage would happen to me. Argh, it's such a cliché, my apologies. But genuinely, I didn't. No one in my family has lost a baby through miscarriage, and it was a fact (in my head alone) that it was a genetic predisposition; also I believed – and please don't laugh – that I had good childbearing hips, and therefore nothing like that could ever happen to me. But it did. Three times.

Now I will be honest and tell you that I had had two children at this point, so my reasons for thinking this way were perhaps justified. Those first times had been so easy and trouble-free that there seemed no reason to worry. So when we tried for that desperately wanted third child, and I was pregnant within three months, I told everyone confidently as soon as the stick showed the all-important blue lines.

However, a week later, after a day of stomach cramps and bleeding, I realised that this was not meant to be. My most vivid memory of this time was being with a nurse who asked how I was feeling. 'OK,' I answered sadly, 'but I just think it would be for the best if I got pregnant straight away. I just feel like I need to be.'

She shook her head at me. 'Respectfully,' she said, 'I don't think that would be the best thing for you. Not at all.'

Oh. I just shrugged at her and left it alone. She was a professional. She dealt with women like me every day. So why did I feel like she'd punched me in my already sore gut? This was definitely a moment that stood out for me. I respect professionals, I really do. But can a statement like that be the answer for everybody? In this case, it didn't feel like the answer for me. I went home and thought about it, and honestly, my feelings didn't change. Yes, my body would need to heal for the recommended six weeks; yes, I would need to grieve; yes, I would need to spend time with my husband and boys to make sure we were doing the right thing; but under all of that I still had the overwhelming urge to be pregnant AS SOON AS POSSIBLE. So it was a happy surprise when, two months or so later, I found I was pregnant again. I felt as though I could breathe, as though someone had taken the vice off my chest. 'Yes! I can still do it! Phew!' I was nervous for the first few weeks, naturally.

Every time I went to the toilet, it was with a sense of trepidation. I still told people pretty much straight away again. First of all, I am not a great believer in keeping it a secret for 12 weeks. When I lost my first baby, it was hard to tell people the bad news, but it would have felt far worse to have kept that life quiet. Second, I am quite rubbish at keeping secrets about myself. But still, it was a quiet celebration. Fast-forward nine months or so and my third baby boy, Jasper, was born, and he was precious, loved and gorgeous. But our family was not to be finished there. We had always wanted four children (and I feel I must stress this because often I get asked if it was because we wanted a girl. A girl would have been wonderful, but I would have celebrated another boy in equal measure), so within a few more years, we considered trying again. Along the way, I miscarried but didn't realise until after the event. Funnily enough, this is often the miscarriage I think about the most – maybe it's the guilt of not ever being aware of his existence until it was over, or maybe it's that this little one never got the positive pregnancy stick. I'm not sure, but little one, fear not, you were loved.

Finally, my last loss came in the form of an ectopic pregnancy, which meant many trips back and forth for tests, injections and scans. It was a tough old season, that one. At one point I was sitting in a waiting room with my husband. We had been hanging around for most of the day, knowing that I was probably going to have treatment to end the pregnancy soon, but waiting for results to confirm it. We were the only ones left; the room gradually dwindling throughout the day as people headed back to their lives. The hospital was in the process of moving their departments around, so the maternity ward was moving to where the early pregnancy assessment unit was, which, of course, led to awkward moments such as this . . . a woman who had recently given birth was shuffling past the waiting room I was in, and following her was a man carrying a car seat with the tiniest, most perfect looking baby girl I'd ever seen. They looked in at us and sat down. I kept my head down to avoid making conversation with them but trust me, I couldn't take my eyes off their baby. The father mumbled something about getting the car then left them. In a small room. With me. I breathed in, and I breathed out, but I couldn't stop the tears welling up in my eyes. It was an incredibly raw and painful moment, but the new mother sitting a few chairs away from me did not need to know this. Within a minute, however, a nurse walked past the room and, after doing a comical double-take (which I could only appreciate a few years later), she gently encouraged the mum to her feet, picked up the precious bundle and walked them out to a more suitable waiting area. Nothing was said, no fuss was made, and for that nurse I am eternally grateful.

I tell you these stories in particular for one reason. I think that our experiences with the professional medical team can leave us reeling or they can leave us feeling buoyed. This experience can be the difference between grieving with anger or grieving with a sense of calm. I appreciate the nurse at the beginning who told me I shouldn't try again as much as I appreciate the nurse who dealt with us so delicately. You see, it gave me a sense that the feeling in my gut should be trusted, that I knew what was best for me and how I needed to deal with my individual loss.

If I could offer one piece of advice, it would be this: the medical professionals do not have to be the aspect that taints your experience. Losing a baby is an awful time, and we all deal with it in our own ways, but these people are here to help us. They know the facts and figures, and all you can do is to go away and trust that they know what they're doing. But don't let their (sometimes ill-offered) opinions get in the way – you know how you feel, so trust that.

Finally, I am grateful to tell you that my story ends well. Almost a year to the date after our loss I went for a routine scan to check how I had recovered physically. They spent some time looking for the small mass which had refused to shrink but which was still of concern. It could not be found on the right side. After some time, this was the conversation. 'OK, then. We can't find the mass; it's completely gone from the right side. However, if anything, there is a small mass on the left side. It's not of concern; it is probably nothing.' I looked at my husband. 'Could it be that I am pregnant?' I asked tentatively. 'We can't answer that . . . if it is then I'm not allowed to say,' and that was that. However, nine months later, my little girl Nell was born, and finally my family was complete and utterly perfect.

Today I am grateful for

DAY 4

Support – Becoming your own health advocate

Whether you have an independent health advocate or not, you still need to be your own health advocate. Speaking up for one's own needs is easy for some, and a real challenge for others. If, like me, you never want to make a fuss or be considered a nuisance, it's easy to stay silent even when the situation dictates that we should speak out. Life will become way better for you if you learn to step out of the box and say, 'When it comes to my health, or my baby's health, I will ask the questions and I will push for answers.' I can assure you that if you are rational and polite with medical people, they will respect your need for information and, in turn, respect you for asking them.

Remember:
- You and your baby deserve the best care possible.
- Tell your story to those who are looking after you, so they can assist you emotionally as well as physically.

- Asking for help or advice is not you being weak or a nuisance, it is you being strong and knowing what you need.
- It is OK to ask to switch doctors or midwives; it is vital you have a good and trusting relationship with the people who are taking care of you.
- If you need information to be repeated do not be afraid to ask; when you are under stress it can be hard to retain information or absorb what is being told to you.
- If you want a second opinion on something, ask for it.
- In the UK you can choose which hospital or GP you get treatment from, so if you would prefer to be seen or treated at an alternative location, just ask.
- Don't be afraid to complain if you received inferior care; the NHS have systems set up to make this process as simple as possible.
- Tell those who are looking after you what you need – if you need more reassurance, explanations, appointments, whatever it is, tell them, as they should be able to help you.

You have the right to be treated with respect and compassion at all times, so don't settle for uncompassionate care, you deserve better than that.

Today I am grateful for

DAY 5

Journalling your pregnancy

What gestation is your baby today? _____

How big are they? _____

What symptoms are you now feeling?

What do you want to remember about how you are feeling
or what you are experiencing?

· ·

The things that you call scars are
what I call my strength.

What you consider to be my undoing
was in fact my hope rising.

What you saw as the end was in fact
the most beautiful beginning.

· · · · · · · · · · · · ZOË CLARK-COATES · · · · · · · · · · · ·

Today I am grateful for

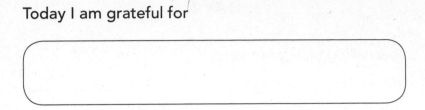

DAY 6

Support – Not feeling able to enjoy pregnancy

When you so desperately want to enjoy something but feel unable to, it's incredibly frustrating. Let me assure you that most people don't enjoy pregnancy 100 per cent of the time, even if they have not lost a baby before. I think the secret of a happy pregnancy rests in just enjoying as many moments as possible – it doesn't have to be all or nothing. Find and welcome the good moments when they happen.

So how can a person discover that enjoyment if it's missing?

Try to find one or two things every day that you like about pregnancy; maybe it's simply the knowledge that you are growing life within. Maybe you enjoy watching your body transform. There are hundreds of moments you may be able to identify as joy-bringers, and focusing on these can make your pregnancy a lot more pleasurable.

However, at times people find it impossible to enjoy pregnancy, and you know what? That is totally OK. You don't need to feel an ounce of guilt if you dislike being pregnant, or hate being pregnant. This has no bearing on how you feel about your baby. Pregnancy is purely the journey to having something you so desperately want: a child.

Today I am grateful for

[ ]

DAY 7

Journal

If someone gave you a magic wand and you could banish one emotion forever, what would it be? Think carefully about this one, as there are big consequences to banishing any emotion from your life.

[ ]

· ·

The pool in front of me was created from tears,
the mountain behind me was made from my fears.

· · · · · · · · · · · · · ZOË CLARK-COATES · · · · · · · · · · · · ·

Today I am grateful for

[ ]

WEEK 20

• •

DAY 1

Support – Insecurity

I never realised how upsetting it could be to lose friends on
Facebook or Instagram until it happened to me. I have a lot of
friends, proper friends, the kind I can call up at 2am, so why
on earth should it bother me if someone has a cull of their
social media friends list and I don't make the cut? I guess it
comes down to insecurity, and that's something I didn't think
I suffered with. I worry I may have done something, or said
something that offended, and I can't help but stew over it.
Since when did I let social media have this sort of control
over my sense of value? And why would I automatically
assume that if we aren't friends on a digital platform, that
means we aren't friends in the real world? Who knows . . .
Maybe you can relate to this? Perhaps you can't? Whether
you can relate or not, there is always something that makes
a person feel insecure.

The issue is we all create our own story in our heads to
make sense of the circumstances in front of us. So for instance
– you cross the street and don't say hello to me. The story I
tell myself is, 'Wow, she must dislike me and want to avoid
me, as she didn't even say hi.' The truth is you didn't even
see me, and you rushed across the road to get to the post
office before it closed. The problem is we often create our
own dialogue and stories around the snippets of information
we see. If one feels any insecurity or rejection, the stories
often feed into that. So what can we do about this? We have
to remind ourselves that the actions of others rarely have
anything to do with us, and everything to do with them,
which is why we shouldn't depend on others to make us feel

secure or loved. We need to avoid obtaining our self-worth from social media likes, follows and comments, as this world can be so fickle and not representative of real life. We need to be aware that the stories and beliefs we create and carry are often completely off the mark, and the only way to be sure of what people think and believe is to ask people directly. Finally, we need to build and work on our personal self-confidence, and ensure we aren't allowing external influences to become our internal voices.

Today I am grateful for

DAY 2

Task

Take one hour to do something you love. Whether that be a soak in the bath and reading a book, a walk in the park, or baking cookies – do it, enjoy it and try to be in the moment – no phones allowed!

Today I am grateful for

DAY 3

Dr Jessica Farren MA, MBBS, MRCOG, PhD, OBGYN

As I have lost one baby am I more likely to lose more?

After one miscarriage or later loss, you are still far more likely to have an uncomplicated pregnancy next time around. This is because the highest likelihood is that what happened was the result of out-of-the-blue 'bad luck' – a chance misfiring of the assembly of chromosomes, or an infection – and is no more likely to happen to you again than to any other woman.

If a cause was found for your pregnancy loss, or losses (usually only the case if you are offered investigations for a later loss, or three or more consecutive losses), then your doctor will have a detailed conversation with you explaining any risks for the future, and what can be done to reduce these risks.

Are there ways to prevent loss?

The majority of losses are the result of genetic abnormalities in the pregnancy that take place in the very first cell divisions. Sadly, this means it could not form a healthy baby, and therefore there is nothing that could be done to prevent it from happening.

In women in whom a cause for losses has been found (usually this is only the case when women have had recurrent miscarriages – three or more – or a loss after the first trimester), sometimes treatment can be offered. For example, women who have had losses explained by a shortening or weakness of the neck of the womb may be offered a stitch in their cervix to prevent it from shortening in a subsequent pregnancy. Women who are more prone to forming blood clots, such as those with a condition known as antiphospholipid syndrome, may benefit from treatment with aspirin and/or heparin injections.

It is important to say that, without test results specifically indicating that there may be issues with the way the woman's blood clots, aspirin has not been shown to have any positive effect and may even increase the risk of miscarriage.

Women often ask whether there is any value in progesterone supplementation, and many women from abroad will have been routinely started on this. However, we have been able in the UK to run the two largest, high-quality studies on progesterone supplementation in women with previous miscarriage, or women with bleeding, and, although there is no evidence for progesterone doing any harm, there is no evidence at present for it conferring any benefit in the vast majority of cases. It is, therefore, not generally available through NHS care.

How can I get my doctor to be more empathetic?

As a doctor, I really hope you won't have cause to ask this question – and I hope that everyone you meet has masses of empathy for anyone who has previously been through loss.

Sadly, sometimes doctors can be accused of getting blasé about miscarriage – because, in truth, up to half of their patients will have been through it, and so they start to view it as an almost normal part of life. They may justify this in the knowledge that certainly some women do not seem to be adversely affected by miscarriage (though if we stopped to think about it, we would realise that just because they don't seem to be affected on the surface, they may still be underneath).

I think the best approach in these situations is simply to explain what you have been through – pointing out why it has affected the way you feel in this pregnancy. If you are struggling with anxiety, be honest about it – and ask them what they would suggest to help you manage it.

Today I am grateful for

DAY 4

Support – Why am I crying all the time?

Some people are more in touch with their emotions than others, and that's just how they are made, but pregnancy is well known for making people shed a regular tear. It is not surprising given the enormous hormonal surges and changes in one's body. Pregnancy is not just about physical changes – it's a mammoth mental and emotional transformation, and we need to give ourselves space and time to adjust.

When you are growing a human, you can either feel like you are more authentically yourself than ever before, or you can feel the exact opposite and lose all sense of who you are. Whichever you are experiencing, know that pregnancy allows everyone the opportunity to ask themselves big life questions. It's OK if this leads you to make changes in your life ahead of your family expanding. Some people use this time to re-evaluate their careers, their hobbies and so much more. When your little one arrives it really could be a new beginning for you all.

So my advice is to try to get comfortable with showing your emotions – tears are a sign of strength, not of weakness. The more you get comfortable with the world witnessing your feelings, the freer you become!

Today I am grateful for

DAY 5

Journalling your pregnancy

What gestation is your baby today? _____

How big are they? _____

What symptoms are you now feeling?

What do you want to remember about how you are feeling or what you are experiencing?

> The issue is if you learn
> to carry your grief internally,
> with very little showing externally,
> people no longer believe
> you are grieving.

ZOË CLARK-COATES

Today I am grateful for

```

```

DAY 6

Support – Health worries and health phobias

My first question would be, did you suffer from worries about your health before you encountered grief and loss? If the answer is 'yes', then you need to try to discover when it started and what triggered it. For the purposes of this section, I am presuming that your health worries started after experiencing baby loss. Grief is well known for doing this; it is partly due to loss revealing a secret trap door beneath your feet: once you know it is there, you fear it will open again without warning. Another reason is that fear sneakily enters people's lives at the point grief enters, and it can attach itself to anything and everything. For some it attaches to leaving the house, or driving, and for many it attaches to worry about health.

So how does a person deal with health fears?

The best way to deal with this is therapy and getting help to switch off the fear, but there are other things you can do. Here is one of my keys to unlocking worry:

- Firstly, just telling yourself not to worry doesn't help, as when you say to the brain not to go to a particular place, it becomes all rebellious and thinks of little else. So I never encourage creating 'no-go places'.
- If you worry, you worry – but once you have permitted yourself to think something, it loses its power to control you. So I say, 'OK brain, you can think of this worry, but I'm not giving it lots of my time.' I will note that the worry is present, and choose to change my thought. I will then do a dramatic right turn in my thought process and think of something completely different.
- Believe me, your brain will encourage you to head straight back to the worry, and this is where you have the power to choose.
- The more you practise turning your thoughts away from fear, the better you will become at it. Eventually, the worry becomes less prominent, and at times it can even vanish completely, as you have starved the fear of all oxygen!

Today I am grateful for

DAY 7

Journal

As a child, what was your biggest love? Do you still love doing it? Perhaps it is time to give it a go or spend more time doing it.

> If we prevent ourselves from feeling the pain,
> we lose the ability to experience the joy.
>
> ZOË CLARK-COATES

Today I am grateful for

WEEK 21

• •

DAY 1

Support – What if . . .

Fear has a typical sentence it likes to throw at people, and whenever I hear it in my brain, I know it is terror talking:
'What if . . . ?'
I know any thought that begins 'What if . . . ?' is fear and worry trying to make me panic.
What if this happens?
What if that takes place?
What if I don't feel that?
Fear is not very creative, it nearly always uses the same language, but that's super-helpful when you want to identify what is behind your thought processes.
So how does one stop it?
The first step in stopping this fear-based thinking is identifying it. Take a note every time you think 'what if'. Then step back and consider: 'What do I want?' Not 'What does anxiety want?' With work (and sometimes help), you can choose to take back your life, and this is where your freedom lies.

Today I am grateful for

┌───┐
│   │
│   │
│   │
└───┘

DAY 2

Task

What advice would you give to a friend who is pregnant following loss? Consider whether you are practising this advice yourself.

Today I am grateful for

Emily's Story

When I saw the second line on the pregnancy stick, I did not feel joy and excitement; I felt fear and dread. When I told my husband, his response was, 'OK, well, here we go again,' and I couldn't have agreed with his comment more, that just about summed it up.

After experiencing two losses, I found being pregnant again terrifying. I felt all-consumed with fear, and then angry that my miscarriages had robbed me of the joy of pregnancy.

Throughout my pregnancy sickness, people often said, 'It'll all be worth it.' I just thought, 'Well, it wasn't the previous times.' I was terrified of going to the loo in case I saw red, terrified of every twinge, every ache or even of feeling less sick! I presumed the panic would be less after the 12-week scan, but it wasn't, the fear was just as intense.

After the scan people would talk about my baby's arrival as a sure thing, but to me, I had a 100 per cent success rate in my babies dying – what proof did they have that this one would be different? I had pregnancy insomnia from week 17 due to anxiety. I was constantly checking and mentally recording the baby's movements, which is exhausting and put me in a constant state of worry, tension and panic.

My two pieces of advice would be:

1. Tell everyone you would want to rally around you if the worst were to happen, as early as you want. We told people as early as four weeks pregnant; we were just desperate for support from our closest friends and family.

2. If you need medical reassurance, get it. Pre-movements, ask for reassurance scans; I think I had four in addition to the standard scans. Hopefully the staff will be kind and compassionate; if not, I stated how my anxiety about my pregnancy had a severe impact upon my mental health, and this seemed to work. Once you can feel movements, it is reassuring to feel the kicks, but for me, this also came with added pressure to be counting them/spotting any changes. If you aren't sure, go in and be monitored. I went in for this at least three times, and the staff were always supportive. However, if yours aren't, I would recommend asking for a different professional.

I did give birth to a beautiful, healthy little girl we've named Alyvia. I fully and wholeheartedly grasp how lucky and blessed we are. However, it did take both my husband and me four months before we truly believed that we would get to keep her and watch her grow up; we didn't dare talk about her as a teen or adult, just in case she never made it.

The new fear of cot death or other complications was sometimes all-consuming – we once visited A&E only to be told she was 'a perfect picture of health'. The anxiety was sky-high. We chose to speak to our GP who was lovely, and we have both been prescribed anti-anxiety medication which has helped. We have also practised meditation, using an app on our phones, put exercise into our routines (gym for my husband and yoga for me) and have taken part in counselling to manage our anxiety. My husband also got CBT (cognitive behavioural therapy) free on the NHS.

Talking to our doctor was the best thing we did. I don't think you can overestimate the huge impact loss can have on subsequent pregnancies and your mental health. Having an open and continuing conversation with my partner as well as with trusted friends and family members has been essential to my grief journey. Just because you have a healthy baby in your arms it doesn't take away all the pain and trauma of baby loss. In fact, for me, it was like all the pent-up emotion of the nine months of terrifying pregnancy, and the two-and-a-half-year pain-filled journey to have a child of our own, all came out.

My children died; I don't believe a human being was designed to be able to cope with that amount of pain. I've accepted it will take time, and I will need help to process what I have been through and will continually have as part of my life's story.

Alyvia is my absolute world; she has brought so much joy and hope into where there was only pain and trauma . . . but my first two children were my whole world too. That doesn't disappear just because Alyvia survived, and I wouldn't want it to. My first two children changed me; their loss was a devastating outcome, undeserved, unfair and unjust; it will never be OK that they died. However, the impact they have had on my life has been huge, both good and bad. They will always be my first two children and Alyvia's older siblings. I am so very grateful that they existed, even if their time was short.

Today I am grateful for

DAY 4

Support – How on earth can I survive another six months of this?

Nine months can feel like an eternity when you are waiting for something you so desperately want, and that's not even taking into account any physical or mental health challenges you may be encountering. But I promise you can survive this journey. Look how far you have already travelled. If you think back to that moment you found out you were pregnant, you had no clue how you would make it to this point – and look, you made it! I assure you when you get to the end of this pregnancy you will look back in awe at all you overcame and achieved. So hold on in there, you can do this.

Add in your name here and repeat it to yourself whenever you need a reminder that you have the strength.

_____, *you have the power to do this. You were born for this moment.*

Whenever you have thought something was unobtainable, you have found a way to achieve it.

Where you thought you were weak, you were in fact strong.

Where you thought you couldn't survive, you have in fact flourished.

You will do this for you.

You will do this for them.

And one day soon, you will say, 'I made it across the finish line, and I ran the race well'.

Today I am grateful for

DAY 5

Journalling your pregnancy

What gestation is your baby today? _____

How big are they? _____

What symptoms are you now feeling?

What do you want to remember about how you are feeling or what you are experiencing?

When you allow yourself to believe
that a good thing may happen
you are allowing those seeds of faith
to bloom into hope.

ZOË CLARK-COATES

Today I am grateful for

DAY 6

Support – Feeling guilt

There is a lot to feel guilty about in this world. Some things we are responsible for, but there is also an awful lot that isn't our responsibility at all. I have learnt that being a parent brings with it a billion guilt trips. I think this is mostly because we want to protect our children from everything and anything, and as this isn't humanly possible (and even if it was it wouldn't be the right thing to do), we carry the guilt. I don't think it's possible to turn off all unnecessary guilt, as that is what makes us human and we often carry baggage that isn't ours to shoulder.

So how does one stop guilt tormenting the mind?

If you are feeling guilt about a situation, you must look at all the information and facts, without fear and emotion, and ascertain whether or not you are responsible. If you discover you are not to blame, you must refuse to listen to that inner voice that wants you to carry false responsibility and shame. You get assertive and say, 'No, this is not my fault, and I refuse to feel responsible.' Eventually (and sometimes after seeking help), the guilt will stop knocking on your door, begging you to carry its weight.

If, after carefully considering whether you are responsible for something happening, you determine you are responsible for an outcome, you need to try to forgive yourself, so you can move forward in life. Some people find they can only find peace after seeking professional help from a therapist, while others are able to work through their feelings on their own.

Be alert to the fact that sometimes other people may try to get you to carry false responsibilities and guilt. This behaviour may stem from their own guilt or issues, or it may be they just want someone to blame, and they picked you. In this situation you have to boldly say, 'No, this is not my responsibility to carry, and I refuse to hold it.' It can take real courage to do this. At times people choose to make this decision internally, without confronting their accuser, but if you are able to have the conversation with them in a constructive manner, it can prevent it happening again.

Just be acutely aware that as you are human, you are going to mess up, you are going to do things you aren't proud of, things you would rather erase from history. So try not to carry the responsibility for those situations that have nothing to do with you.

Today I am grateful for

DAY 7

Journal

What does your inner voice say to you most? Can you make this voice more positive?

. . . .

Fear's plan is to make you so scared of
drowning that you don't even try to swim.

The issue . . .

You may just end up sinking,
so refuse to listen to its voice!

. . . . ZOË CLARK-COATES . . . .

Today I am grateful for

WEEK 22

DAY 1

Support – When people tell you not to dwell on a previous loss

It makes me so angry when I hear someone say a baby loss shouldn't be dwelt on. Still, I try to imagine that the person saying it has a good heart and either has issues understanding loss, or personal issues that stop them being empathetic and compassionate.

Let me reassure you, whenever you think about the baby you lost (or any other person you have lost), you are not dwelling or being maudlin. You are thinking about a person you loved (and still love) and will always treasure. They are as much a part of your future as they were a part of your past, and it's very healthy to talk about them. I worry more for those who feel unable to talk about the ones they have lost than for those who feel the freedom to be open, as that is often down to an underlying issue.

So how does a person handle this sort of comment? Well, I guess it depends on who said it. Do you have an ongoing relationship with them? If the answer is yes, I would say if you feel able to address the comment and want to, then do. If it's not someone you are in a regular relationship with, and perhaps you don't even care what their opinion is, then decide on whether it's worth your time even addressing it. Pick your battles and conserve your energy for the things you have to face head-on.

If you decide you do need to address an inconsiderate comment, I encourage you to do it sensitively – even though this may not be deserved. I understand that, in the heat of emotion, you may not care about being kind, as someone just deeply hurt you. But if you want to encourage a change of attitude and perception at their end, the best way to do that is to avoid putting them on the defensive or, worse, on the attack. If you can be full of grace and choose your words well, you have the chance to make a difference, not just for you, but potentially for other people too.

Be prepared that even the best-reasoned argument may fall on deaf ears, and some people will never change their views or beliefs, however much they are proved wrong. If you encounter this attitude, you may need to reluctantly accept that you made your point, and will have to leave it at that. You cannot force change, and you can't argue with someone who has no intention of either listening to you or viewing things differently. But you do have the right to set a new boundary line and say, 'Whether you agree with me or not, I will not permit you to say this to me again. If you do, it will affect our relationship.' If a person can't respect a boundary line laid by someone else, it says a lot about them, and you will then have to choose how you move the relationship forward.

Today I am grateful for

DAY 2

Task

What have you been postponing until you feel ready? This may be to do with your pregnancy or perhaps something totally unrelated.

Do you think you could take a chance and just move forward? Now may not be the right time of course, but maybe it is? Stepping out of your comfort zone always takes courage, but you are often rewarded for moving forwards into the unknown.

Make a list of tasks you have been postponing:

Today I am grateful for

DAY 3

Clare Bourne MCSP, MHCPC, MPOGP, Pelvic Health Physiotherapist

Why do people suffer from pelvic pain when pregnant?

Pelvic girdle pain can occur for a variety of reasons. It is often a combination of factors rather than an individual one. Possible reasons are the pelvic joints moving asymmetrically, muscle imbalances around the pelvis, weaker core muscles, including the abdominal, gluteal and pelvic floor muscles. Change of posture can also have an impact. Hormone changes can play a part, but this is often not as significant as the other factors mentioned above.

What can people do to help relieve pelvic pain?

First of all, know that pelvic pain can be treated, and early assessment and treatment can really help outcomes and pain. Therefore, as soon as you have symptoms, ask for a referral from either your midwife or GP to your local women's health or pelvic health physiotherapy service for assessment, treatment and support. In the meantime, the following day-to-day tips can really help manage symptoms:

- *Sit down for activities like putting on trousers, to prevent standing on one leg.*
- *Keep your knees together for movements such as rolling in bed and standing up, and squeeze your knees together and your bottom muscles when standing up.*
- *Use a plastic bag on your car seat to help you get in and out easily.*

- *Keep active within pain-free ranges. It is important to note this during and after the activity. Sometimes the aggravating movement doesn't create pain straight away.*
- *Use a rucksack instead of a one-shoulder bag, especially if carrying heavy laptops etc.*
- *Reduce your stride length in walking – sounds small but can make a huge difference.*
- *Often working on exercises to strengthen the bottom (gluteal) muscles and deep core is better than walking if you suffer from pelvic pain.*
- *Try not to sit cross-legged, even if it doesn't create pain at the time.*

There is a great leaflet by Pelvic Obstetric Gynaecological Physiotherapy (POGP), a professional network affiliated to the Chartered Society of Physiotherapy, called Pregnancy-Related Pelvic Girdle Pain *which you can access for free on the internet.*

Why do people suffer from back pain while pregnant?

Pelvic pain can present in the lower back area so it can be hard to know whether it is your back or pelvis that is causing the pain. Some pregnant women have pain originating from the lower segments of the spine, known as the lumbar spine. The pain can be coming from the joints or the surrounding muscles, and for some the nerves.

The most common driver is the change in posture around the spine and pelvis during pregnancy. The pelvis tilts forwards, and the lower spine increases its curve forwards. Additionally, women often have weaker core muscles, as mentioned previously, which also means the support around the spine is reduced and can cause other muscles to become tighter as they compensate for the weaker muscles.

What can people do to relieve back pain?

Again treatment and early referral are best; it is not a part of pregnancy you should have to accept as normal. For most women, gentle movement around the back will help symptoms. Exercises like pelvic tilts or cat/camel (which you may have done during yoga or Pilates) are great places to start. Working on the movement of your upper back is often very beneficial as well. Think about your sitting posture, especially if you work at a desk a lot. My top tip is to take an old towel, tape it into a sausage shape and sit with this behind your lower back; it provides a lot of support and helps keep the natural posture of the spine. Additionally, a warm water bottle on the lower back at the end of the day can help ease any muscle tension. Pregnancy Pilates is a great form of exercise if you are experiencing some back pain as it focuses on strengthening and movement, which most women find incredibly beneficial.

If you have back pain with pain down the legs, I would highly advise seeing a physiotherapist before starting any exercises for some further, and specific, advice as treatment can be different.

Why are pelvic floor muscle exercises important in pregnancy?

The pelvic floor muscles, which sit at the bottom of the pelvis, lengthen during pregnancy and weaken from the weight of the baby sitting on them. Exercising your pelvic floor helps to maintain strength and also prevent symptoms of urinary leakage, which some women will report during pregnancy, especially towards the end. It can also help your postnatal recovery. They are so easy to forget, but I recommend trying to associate them with something, like mealtimes, or set a phone reminder, or there is a great NHS app called the Squeezy App that you can use to jog your memory. Pelvic floor exercises are really for life, but pregnancy is a time when we need to give the muscles a little extra TLC.

Why do some women leak urine either during or after pregnancy, and what can I do to resolve it?

Urinary leakage can occur for a variety of reasons, but for lots of women, it is caused by weak pelvic floor muscles as mentioned above. Pelvic floor muscle exercises are therefore often the answer, but lots of us don't know how to do them correctly. The best cues to think of are first holding wind, and then adding on holding urine, as you exhale, then fully relaxing the muscles again before the next contraction. You can do them lying down, sitting or standing. It can be really hard to know if you are doing them correctly and, therefore, I advise asking for a referral to your local women's health physiotherapy service for assessment and support. Again, it is so treatable and isn't something to suffer with in silence.

Today I am grateful for

DAY 4

Support – Waiting for test results

Waiting for test results is obviously going to be a stressful time when all you want to hear is an instant 'everything is fine'. Your imagination is not going to be your best friend when you have to sit and wait. So what can you do to make this time easier? My best tip is to keep busy. Throw yourself into as many activities as possible, whether they be physical or mental ones – the less time you give yourself to imagine the worst, the better. No worry will change the result; all you will do is make yourself feel drained emotionally, so try not to let your mind take you to dark places. My policy was to allow myself to dwell only on positive thoughts unless I was given sufficient evidence I should think otherwise. So while I waited for results, I kept telling myself everything was great. Of course, there were times when my brain told me it wasn't, and my fight-or-flight response went on high alert, but through intense practice, I was able to keep my mind in a state of positivity a lot of the time.

Due to my medical history, my medical team were really sensitive around these times and would do everything they could to rush test results. They also agreed to call me the moment results were in, and this really helped me, so definitely request this with your team.

I feel I do need to disclose that there was one test we had to wait a few days to hear back from, and it was one of the most challenging periods of my life. I didn't cope well and basically took to my bed. I was physically ill myself at the time, recovering from surgery, and the only option seemed to hide away. My duvet became my safety blanket, and even though every minute felt like an hour, I survived it. If you have a wait like this, you will survive it too.

Let me also remind you about this wonderful website which may help you: https://www.thewaitingroom.life/

Today I am grateful for

DAY 5

Journalling your pregnancy

What gestation is your baby today? _____

How big are they? _____

What symptoms are you now feeling?

What do you want to remember about how you are feeling or what you are experiencing?

The world is often screaming,
'What do you need?'
The answer is often:
Time to feel. Time to heal.

ZOË CLARK-COATES

Today I am grateful for

DAY 6

Task

How I loved picking names! I have always loved looking at name meanings and thoroughly enjoyed deciding on our children's names. We named every one of our babies, those who ran ahead and those who stayed, as we believe every person deserves a name.

We bought a couple of name books, and highlighted all the names we loved. We even used different coloured highlighters, to determine what would be an excellent first name, and what we liked as middle names. The girls love looking at these books now and seeing all their potential names.

Both Esmé and Brontë have declaration middle names that mean something profound to us, and we felt this was important given our journey to have them.

Esmé's full name is Esmé Emilia Promise – the meaning of her name is *Much loved, Soft spirited, Promise*. We settled on the name Promise because we believed wholeheartedly that we would have a child to raise one day, and when Esmé was born we saw this dream become a reality. She was the long-held promise that we had hoped for through years of pain.

Brontë's full name is Brontë Jemima Hope. Her name means *Bestower of Peace and Hope*. My pregnancy was fraught with illness, danger and fear, but through it all we prayed for peace, and held on to the hope that she would survive and thrive, which is how we settled on her name.

Thankfully Andy and I have similar tastes when it comes to names, so we never disagreed – but we had to both love them for them to stay on the potential list. By the time the girls were both six months' gestation their names were picked and selected. We chose not to tell anyone the names (not even immediate family) until after they were born, as we wanted them to be a surprise, and didn't want people to put us off our choices.

What name, or names, are you considering?

Today I am grateful for

DAY 7

Journal

What makes you feel out of control?

If you dislike feeling out of control, can you identify why?

What can you do to help yourself feel more in control?

Our lost children are not pain,
they are not a wound,
they are not a trauma.
The loss is the agony, not the precious
soul that was taken too soon.
So when people say,
'Maybe it's best not to talk about
them in case you reopen a wound',
they are simply not understanding
that our children are a gift.
They are a beautiful treasure
people spend their life searching for.
By talking about them, we heal.
By sharing their story,
however short it may have been,
we cast a light in someone else's dark world.
And, perhaps most importantly, we are acknowledging
they were here,
that their lives made a difference,
that because they existed we are different,
that because of them,
the world is a better place.

ZOË CLARK-COATES

Today I am grateful for

WEEK 23

● ●

DAY 1

Support – The constant need for the loo

Boy did no one prepare me for this . . . Let me tell you, before pregnancy, I was often called a human camel due to my ability to hold needing the loo. I have always hated using public restrooms so this skill was a real blessing. Once I needed the bathroom as I left the house, held it for the journey to the airport, decided when I was there to wait until I got on the plane. On the flight I thought, *I am going to try to hold it until I land.* Eight hours later I got off that plane and thought, *I think I can hold it until I get to the hotel in New York.* You know what (get ready to applaud), I made it! I feel this deserves some kind of award; I don't know what type, but it's impressive, right? (And no, I didn't get a urinary tract infection!) Then I got pregnant. It was like my bladder was punishing me for making it hold it so often in the past; I spent my life searching out restrooms wherever I visited.

The reason you have an increased need to urinate when pregnant is not only due to having a baby bouncing on your bladder, it's also due to the hormones. There were times I seriously considered setting up my office desk in the loo; in fact, I even considered moving the bed into the bathroom at one point, as I seemed to spend every night walking back and forth to the loo, rather than sleeping.

So why am I telling you this . . . ? Well, one, I wanted to tell you about the award I am still waiting to receive, and two, I wanted to reassure you that for me this constant need to urinate stopped the moment the baby was born, and I would have loved for someone to tell me that your bladder often returns to normal post-delivery.

I do want to encourage you to do your pelvic floor exercises every day though, as you will be mightily rewarded once you deliver your little one if that muscle is strong. I suggest printing the exercise tips your midwife will give you and sticking them to the back of your bathroom door, so you can do them every time you go to the loo. I promise you if you ever decide to become a pro trampoliner and enter the Olympics you will thank me for this tip. Heck, you may also thank me the first time you have a sneezing episode as that's when you know if you have a good strong pelvic floor!

Today I am grateful for

DAY 2

Task

Is there anything you would like to be different after you have had your baby? Would you like to change jobs? Find a new hobby? Start to process something to do with your childhood? Write a list and if you are able to put any of these things into action now, why not make a start.

_____

_____

_____

_____

_____

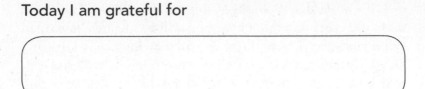

DAY 3

Rachel's Story

When we fell pregnant with our second baby it was quite a surprise: after trying for our first for nearly two years we were expecting a similar journey, but after only a few months we had that positive test. Everything was great, I'd had my booking-in appointment, had my 12-week scan date, and we were looking forward to the future.

The day before my scan I started spotting; I immediately called maternity triage. As my scan was the next day I was told just to monitor things and if it became heavy or painful to call back. The next 24 hours felt like forever. We eventually made it to the hospital for the scan; thankfully it was scheduled for the early morning. Unfortunately, the scan showed that the baby had stopped developing, and they attributed the spotting to my body starting to recognise this. We went home in tears, having to walk past several excited parents-to-be waiting for their own scans, and I miscarried naturally the next day.

Nervously we started trying to conceive almost as soon as my body had recovered from the pregnancy, but this took time. After a year, I was referred to the fertility clinic, and just after this I found out I was pregnant again. Unfortunately, I also miscarried this baby in early pregnancy. The consultant allowed us to carry on with our referral due to miscarrying again and I began regular blood testing and ultrasounds: I was then diagnosed with polycystic ovary syndrome, or PCOS. This possibly explained the miscarriages and the difficulty conceiving, as I only ovulate a few times a year.

I was just about to start my first cycle with Clomid when I discovered I was pregnant again. We had recently moved across the country and had been preoccupied with removals and unpacking, so I hadn't taken any notice that I was late. At first, we were excited that it had happened without any help, but then I was scared I would miscarry again. I was constantly looking up symptoms and other people's experiences online, looking for something similar to show me that everything would be OK this time. I reluctantly arranged my booking-in appointment. Unfortunately, my new NHS Trust wouldn't let me have an early scan, despite my having had two previous miscarriages, and this put me on edge a bit as it was such a long wait until my 12-week scan. I didn't want a repeat of what happened with our second pregnancy.

We decided to pay for a private scan, despite how expensive it was – we just needed to know if everything was OK. The two-week wait for the scan felt like a year. On the morning of it my stomach was doing somersaults and I felt sick. I wasn't able to eat anything and had to force a bottle of water down so I'd have a full bladder. The ladies couldn't have been kinder, doing everything they could to put us at ease, understanding about our history. I could barely breathe the moment the sonographer placed the Doppler on my abdomen, just praying over and over in my head she'd find something, anything. After a few moments there it was, the tiny heartbeat flickering away; she reassured us that everything looked perfect. I burst into tears; it was such a relief.

We immediately told close family: it felt like if we talked about him/her, then it made it more real and everything would be OK.

The following few weeks until my 12-week scan were a bit nerve-racking; despite having had the early scan I had a niggling doubt that it was all going to come crashing down again. I just needed to get past that 12-week mark.

In between this, I had my booking-in appointment. The midwife was very matter-of-fact, writing down and discussing my two angels as if it was something that happened all the time, like popping to the shop for a pint of milk, barely interested in the early scan photographs I took along with me. She was pleasant enough, but it made me nervous about the next few weeks' wait. It was a nice feeling walking out with my handheld notes, though: written proof on my medical record that I was indeed pregnant again. I never got this far with my last pregnancy.

I'd started feeling odd twinges here and there; I would panic each time, but looking back these were just implantation and growing pains. I stopped going to the gym, running up and down the stairs, doing anything that I thought could remotely harm the baby. This one I was going to try my best to keep safe. I know it was likely nothing like that would have caused me to miscarry, but I couldn't take that chance.

The day of the 12-week scan arrived. I was nervous all day as it wasn't until after lunch. Thankfully I was busy at work in the morning and my colleague tried her best to keep my mind off it, talking about upcoming meetings. My stomach was in knots on the way to the hospital, and while we sat waiting; it didn't help that the clinic was running late. It was eventually my turn, and the sonographer found the heartbeat immediately. I couldn't stop crying; we'd made it to 12 weeks.

When we had the 20-week scan, I had to go alone as our son had chickenpox so he wasn't at nursery. With no one to distract me all I could think about were things that could be wrong. I hadn't yet felt any movement, so I began to worry about that. Everything was perfectly fine, but it took a long time for the sonographer to get the pictures she needed. This made me nervous when she couldn't get any clear pictures of the heart; even after a walk and a cold drink she still was unable to get them. I was to go back in one to two weeks for a follow-up scan as she'd run out of time. Despite knowing everything was OK it played on my mind constantly – what if there was a heart defect and that was why she couldn't get a good view? I'd also still not felt any movements, but after checking my scan report, I discovered this was because of an anterior placenta cushioning any kicks.

My follow-up scan was two weeks later, and everything was as it should be. I confirmed with the sonographer that my placenta was indeed anterior, and that put me at ease.

The following weeks up to my due date were a mix of being so happy when feeling the baby moving to being worried something else could go wrong. I had to keep telling myself I'd got past both 12- and 20-week scans and they'd have picked up anything wrong. Then I had a few episodes of reduced movements. Thankfully baby had just tucked herself up all comfy and kicked me all night to make up for it.

Once I was in labour, I didn't feel worried at all. We were about to meet her, and all was well. I was more focused on achieving my long-awaited VBAC, which I think helped greatly, diverting my attention.

The moment I got to hold my daughter was one of the greatest moments of my life, and she was worth every sleepless night and panic-filled minute.

Today I am grateful for

DAY 4

Support – Baby movement in the womb

We now live in a society that rightly encourages us to monitor movements to protect our babies, but with that comes this heavy weight of responsibility that, if we don't notice a change in movement, perhaps we are to blame for any issues that arise. When you are already carrying grief and fear, this can make monitoring movement extremely challenging and terrifying. So how do you cope and survive it?

In my case, I tried to establish my baby's pattern early on. I would give myself time each day to notice the movements, and once I had felt them, I kept telling myself all was well. Importantly I also didn't hesitate to reach out to my doctors or midwives if I thought anything felt different or was worrying me. This sounds like an easy thing to do; but it wasn't, as I am from that generation where you don't want to make a fuss, and you don't want to be considered a nuisance, so asking to be monitored did not come naturally to me. Still, I chose to step out of my comfort zone and always asked to be checked for the sake of my baby, and also for the sake of my peace of mind.

Some people get reassurance from counting the number of kicks their baby does each day, but for me, I knew that that was going to make me on edge every minute of every day, so doing two checks a day, one in the morning and one in the evening, seemed OK. I would often have times where I would rub my stomach and beg for the baby within to give me a sign they were all right. Just feeling those movements and kicks made me breathe a sigh of relief. Only those who have encountered loss will understand those waves of panic, when you are terrified that your baby may not be alive, and you just crave immediate reassurance that they are well.

The bottom line is that only you know what is right for you when it comes to monitoring movements, and I would encourage you to be guided by your doctor and midwife on this – they have your back, so lean on them for advice and you will feel so much more secure.

Today I am grateful for

DAY 5

Journalling your pregnancy

What gestation is your baby today? _____

How big are they? _____

What symptoms are you now feeling?

What do you want to remember about how you are feeling
or what you are experiencing?

· ·

People need to be reminded that they
can survive pregnancy post-loss.
It is easy to forget that when stumbling in the darkness.
So let me be the one to remind you today.
You will make it through.
You will find a way to navigate the fear.
You will flourish.
You will survive.
You will do so in honour of the ones you have lost
and because you hold a hope for the ones you will raise.

· · · · · · · · · · · · ZOË CLARK-COATES · · · · · · · · · · · · ·

Today I am grateful for

DAY 6

Support – Heavy heart

Grief can make your heart feel heavy. Loss makes you suddenly aware of the weight of love, of pain, and of missing someone. Does your heart eventually get lighter as time goes on? I don't think it does; I think you just get accustomed to its new weight. The weight it now is is your new normal. It does take time to get used to the new weight, though. For some, it takes months, for others years, and some a lifetime, but you learn to carry it even if you are never comfortable doing so.

The unique thing about having a heavy heart is you learn to recognise others who have one too. You can bond with these people deeply and authentically, as you both know the true value and fragility of life. You are also acutely aware:

- That love and loss are infinitely connected.
- That one never 'gets over loss'.
- That there is no forgetting, just embracing.
- That life continues whether you want it to or not.
- That grief changes you so radically; it can be hard for you to recognise yourself, let alone others recognise you.
- That pain can make you love harder, or love less – you have the choice.

Today I am grateful for

DAY 7

Journal

If you could design the perfect friend, what would they be like? Are you that friend to others?

People told me I was brave not to give up,
but want to know a secret?

I did give up.

We all give up.

When pain is overwhelming,
when fear is all-consuming,
we all scream at the
sky and say, 'Enough!'

But something magical
happens when we quit;
When we say,
'I can't take any more!'

We discover life carries on regardless and,
when we have nothing more
to offer, a new strength is sent
to carry us through.

ZOË CLARK-COATES

Today I am grateful for

WEEK 24

DAY 1

Support – Aches and pains in pregnancy . . . what is normal?

It is so hard to know what is 'normal' in pregnancy, especially post-loss, as you can easily fall into a pattern of overanalysing every single ache and pain. I think one of the questions I asked most when pregnant was, 'Do you think that is normal?' I have personally lived this, so I totally get it, that worry that you are missing a sign or an issue. Firstly, let me reassure you that nine times out of ten noticing or not noticing something wouldn't change the outcome. This knowledge brought me some reassurance, as it lifted a weight off my shoulders. Secondly, anything and everything can ache and feel weird when pregnant. You forget what normal feels like, and pain you would never even notice when you aren't pregnant feels like a huge issue when you are. My best advice is to lean on your doctors and midwives when you are worried. My doctor was able to reassure me that all was well, and the feelings I was having were just a routine part of pregnancy.

The aches that always worried me the most were regular period-type pains. To me, these felt like an impending sign of loss, but they weren't. My doctor told me they were stretching pains, and a sign my baby was growing. So try not to fret. Speak out about your worries and let the medics reassure you.

Today I am grateful for

DAY 2

Task

Write down what you love about pregnancy and what you dislike about pregnancy.

Today I am grateful for

DAY 3

Dr Jessica Farren MA, MBBS, MRCOG, PhD, OBGYN

Can I request extra scans for peace of mind?

Yes, you can. There is even some evidence that supports that medical care, which may include regular ultrasound scans, may be associated with a lower risk of miscarriage. Some units with specialist recurrent miscarriage services can offer clinics where women who have experienced multiple, or late, losses are seen every two to three weeks throughout the first trimester. If you don't have access to such a service, there is no reason why your GP cannot refer you into an early pregnancy unit for a scan (or two) for reassurance.

If you have previously experienced early losses, you are likely to find that, once you start feeling movements, you have the reassurance you need from that – as well as the routine monitoring of the size of your bump, and the standard 20-week scan. If you still feel you would like more scans, you should ask for them. Whether or not the hospital will facilitate this request may depend on their capacity to do so. You may find you wish to supplement what the hospital can offer you with scans that you pay for privately.

If you have previously had a loss later in the second or third trimester, you will usually be booked in for scans to assess the growth of the baby every four weeks. If you have concerns about the baby's movements later in pregnancy, or if your bump is growing at a slower rate than expected, you will usually be referred for a one-off scan at that point.

Can I ask to see a consultant for peace of mind?

Antenatal care in the UK is generally midwifery-led. Women who have experienced a previous later loss (after 13 weeks of pregnancy) will usually automatically be referred to doctor-led, or shared care. This is not usually the case for women who have experienced losses earlier in their pregnancy, although some units will have specialist doctor-led care for women who have had recurrent miscarriages.

If you wish to see a doctor, you should ask your midwife to refer you. You may find they want to understand a little more about the reasons behind the request, to see if they can offer you the peace of mind you need – but you should not have any problem arranging this.

When you are seen in a hospital doctor-led antenatal clinic, you may be seen by a consultant or one of their juniors. It's worth pointing out that these 'juniors' may have many years of training in obstetrics, and always have the support of their consultants – so it is likely to be worth seeing them in the first instance. Of course, if you feel that you are not getting the reassurance you need, or your concerns are not being appropriately responded to, you should have no qualms about asking to see the most senior doctor at that, or a subsequent, appointment.

Can I ask to change doctors?

Yes, you can. If your desire to change doctors is based on a difference of opinions, your doctor should be aware that it is an important part of their professional conduct to respect your right to a second opinion.

You may find the easiest way to go about this is to speak to your midwife, or the maternity booking telephone line in your hospital, and simply ask them to change your subsequent appointment to be under a different team.

Today I am grateful for

DAY 4

Support – When worry is making you think you are going insane

Worry does have the ability to make people think they are losing the plot during pregnancy. If I had a penny for every person who asks me, 'Am I going mad?' I would be rich! Worry is so incessant and unrelenting it can make anyone question their sanity. It's like another person crawled into your brain and won't stop talking, constantly throwing torment into every situation.

The amazing, beautiful, fantastic thing about this is – IT IS POSSIBLE TO FIND FREEDOM FROM WORRY.

- Worry will lie to you and tell you there is no way out.
- Worry will try to convince you that this is just how you are wired.
- Worry will tell you that if you don't worry, bad things will happen, as worry is preventing danger from coming to your door.
- Worry says all of these things, and a whole lot more, because worry is a liar.

- Worry wants to make you feel like you are going mad so it can control you even more.
- When you are worried about the amount you worry, you know it has a grip on you, and it is time to say 'enough'.

If you can ask your doctor for CBT therapy, do it now. Start the process and get help, as your freedom awaits. You don't need to live with this. Worry is like a leech, it sucks all your lifeblood from you, and makes life an ongoing battle. However, with work, life can totally change for the better.

Today I am grateful for

DAY 5

Journalling your pregnancy

What gestation is your baby today? _____

How big are they? _____

What symptoms are you now feeling?

What do you want to remember about how you are feeling or what you are experiencing?

It is OK to be different.
It is OK to be bruised.
It is OK to show one's scars.
I don't know when the world started to tell us
perfection is beautiful, but it is wrong.
The truth is, vulnerability is breath-taking.
Being authentic is inspiring and walking
with our head held high, carrying no
shame from our journey,
is where real beauty can be found.

ZOË CLARK-COATES

Today I am grateful for

DAY 6

Support – Being told you are brave or strong for talking about your lost babies

The term 'brave and strong' is thrown around a lot when people are grieving, and I think most bereaved people will tell you they feel a million miles away from both. You mostly keep going as you have no other choice, and it's hard to believe or accept this is bravery or strength when all you have done is drag yourself out of bed to do the things you were obliged to do.

So are you brave or strong, and am I?

Yes, we probably are, but actually who cares? What's important is that you will survive today. Tomorrow you will try to survive again, and I am confident you will make it, just like I did.

I do think being willing to try again for a baby after loss shows unbelievable tenacity and strength. Knowing you will be holding your breath for nine months takes guts, so I applaud you. And you should be so proud of yourself.

Today I am grateful for

DAY 7

Journal

If you could change one thing about your personality, what would it be?

What character trait are you most proud of having?

Be patient.

Give yourself time to heal.

Rebuilding yourself following heartbreak
and loss is a slow process and it
is not something that can be rushed.

So stop.

Breathe.

Wait.

Process.

Rise.

ZOË CLARK-COATES

Today I am grateful for

WEEK 25

· ·

DAY 1

Support – Fear of sex or intimacy in pregnancy

Fear of sex/intimacy is such a common worry in pregnancy, especially post-loss. For some couples, it is a big issue; for others, it is not a problem at all. I want to encourage you to talk to one another if it's a problem in your relationship, and also to speak to a health professional or counsellor if you feel it would help.

Some don't want to have physical relations as it just doesn't feel right when pregnant; others are terrified that sex may trigger bleeding or loss. If the latter is your concern, your doctor or midwife will be able to reassure you that this is not dangerous, so it is worth being brave and opening up the conversation.

So how do you handle this issue if one party wants sexual intimacy and the other doesn't? Well, this can be tricky whether someone is pregnant or not, but the important thing is no one should be made to feel guilty or pressured into doing anything they don't want. Talking is the key as, once you express your views and opinions, it means your partner will know where you stand.

Today I am grateful for

DAY 2

Task

Has grief or this pregnancy brought past pain or upset to the surface for you? If it has, consider how you could or should deal with it. Do you feel you need professional assistance? Or do you just need to sit and talk with your partner, family member or friend? A helpful exercise can be to write down all the issues that have emerged and see if there is a common thread to them all.

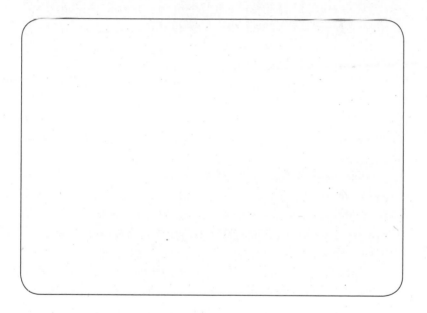

Today I am grateful for

DAY 3

Zoë B's Story

I never thought I'd be writing this piece. Despite knowing the depressing statistics about baby loss, for some reason I didn't think it would happen to us. I have a beautiful three-year-old daughter, and I'm currently 30 weeks pregnant, but this is my fourth pregnancy. I lost two babies between my two girls.

With each blue line, each pregnancy, came the heady mix of fear and excitement – the planning, the birthday-date figuring and the waves of nausea. Tragically two of those babies didn't make it, and I experienced the crushing loss and grief that I suspect you also know so well.

So into the fourth pregnancy, same blue lines, same excitement – but this time tinged with fear. What if it happens again? What then? Looking back, I can see I held my breath for most of the first seven weeks of this pregnancy. That was the line in the sand my mind drew to keep myself safe. It was a form of self-preservation – not to get too attached, not to get too excited. Just in case, I thought.

Eight weeks came, and I started to feel my mind and muscles relax; it felt like a big exhale. Maybe, just maybe this might be the one. I went for a scan at nine weeks, and I remember my heart thudding as the sonographer looked for the heartbeat. It felt like an eternity. The cool, kind but breezy look on her face against my tight jaw and racing mind. 'There it is,' she said as I heard the most welcome sound in the world – our baby's heartbeat.

I rushed out to my husband who was waiting outside with our daughter (we didn't have childcare that day and didn't want her in the room just in case). We both burst into tears. The relief. Since that day I have been focused on relaxing into this pregnancy – as the fears have come up in my mind, the 'what ifs' and maybes, I've used my mindfulness practices to keep myself positive and focused on what I want to happen, not on what I don't.

Every time a fearful or anxious thought has come into my mind I've accepted it and understood why it's there, but kindly reassured myself that thinking the worst only steals the joy of the current moment. Thinking and worrying about the worst-case scenario wouldn't make it any easier to deal with if the worst did happen. I know that from experience.

I use my mindfulness practice to come back to right now – in the present moment, where all is well. As the fearful thoughts try to take hold, I place my hand on my growing belly and breathe in gratitude. As simplistic as it sounds, gratitude is the best antidote I've found to fear and anxiety.

I'm now 30 weeks and looking forward to meeting our little girl. I've found pregnancy after a loss a mental challenge – but one I'm determined to beat.

Today I am grateful for

DAY 4

Support – What if I've eaten something I shouldn't have?

I hear from people regularly who are utterly terrified as they have consumed a food product or beverage that they then discovered they shouldn't have. My first piece of advice to anyone who is worrying about this is to speak to your doctor or midwife if you are at all concerned, as they will hopefully be able to reassure you. Secondly, remember that all food and drink advice is precisely that – advice. It does not mean you have failed or endangered your baby if you accidentally ate some unpasteurised cheese. If you have consumed something either before you knew you were pregnant, or after finding out and are now scared, you need to try to let the worry go. No panic will change the fact you have consumed it; it will just cause you extreme anxiety if you keep worrying about it.

All you can do when you find out you are pregnant is look at the most recent advice on what to and not to consume and do your best to comply. Opinion regularly changes, so it's always worth looking up the latest guidelines, as things that were previously not recommended may now be deemed safe, since new research often changes safety protocols.

Today I am grateful for

DAY 5

Journalling your pregnancy

What gestation is your baby today? _____

How big are they? _____

What symptoms are you now feeling?

What do you want to remember about how you are feeling or what you are experiencing?

. . . .

I can always recognise those who have been broken.

For they now carry a light – a light that can only be bestowed on those who have been shattered by loss.

They are filled with greater levels of compassion, of empathy and of kindness, for they know first-hand what true pain feels like.

. . . . ZOË CLARK-COATES . . . .

Today I am grateful for

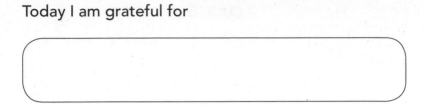

DAY 6

Support – When the reassurance from a doctor or midwife only lasts a few hours

Let me reassure you that it is so common to be back in a state of panic just hours after you've had your fears assuaged by your medical team. You are not going mad.

When you have previously been through a traumatic event, your imagination is not your friend, and fear can often run away with itself. If you heard good news in the past which then went sour, then of course your brain will be sounding off an alarm in your head, and you will be on high alert.

So how do you find peace and, importantly, keep the peace? You talk about your fears with your partner, friends, family and your medical team! The more you speak about and address your worries and concerns, the more peace you will experience.

Initially, I would suggest not setting the bar too high. For instance, it's unrealistic to think, 'From now on, I will not worry at all.' This is just setting yourself up to fail. Try small goals of worrying less or having worry-free periods. By developing healthy habits to control your stress levels, you are helping yourself long term, as these are crucial life skills.

One practical piece of advice for sustained peace following medical appointments is always to take a written list of questions in with you. A lot of anxiety is caused by remembering afterwards queries or worries that you forgot to raise during the appointment. Preparing questions in advance and getting them answered brings real reassurance. I always advise people to keep a notebook specifically for this. Whenever you think of a question, day or night, write it in the notebook, and take this with you to every appointment. I also encourage people to write down the answers they are given so they can go back and reread the answers; this also means they can share that information with their partner or friends and family at a later date.

Today I am grateful for

DAY 7

Journal

How has your most painful moment changed you?

How has your most amazing moment changed you?

· ·

Talk about it.

Then talk some more.

Then a little more.

The story you hold deep in your heart
wants to be told – needs to be told.

It is in the telling.

It is in the sharing.

It is in the revealing of your soul
that true healing and growth begins.

· · · · · · · · · · · · · ZOË CLARK-COATES · · · · · · · · · · · · ·

Today I am grateful for

WEEK 26

• •

DAY 1

Support – When feeling ill makes you fear for your mental health

I don't think we discuss enough the influence sickness and physical illness can have on one's mental health. You don't have to have previously suffered from depression or other mental health conditions to struggle in this area.

If you feel too ill to go about everyday life, it can be extremely challenging emotionally. Likewise, if you always feel nauseous and don't even know what to do with yourself as you feel so deathly, this can play havoc with your mental health. As I mentioned earlier in the book, pregnancy made me very sick, and to go from being physically able to bed-bound was hard. I had no idea if the symptoms would end the following week or in eight months' time. Once you have been sick week after week, month after month, you start to not even be able to imagine the illness ending when the baby is born, as it's hard to look past the 24 hours you are struggling through.

So how can someone survive this?

- Firstly, reach out to your doctors and midwives and explain to them how you are feeling. There may be medications or advice they can offer you to help you through.
- Secondly, tell your friends and family. It's natural to withdraw from the world when you are feeling so poorly, and that can mean you don't have the vital support you need, so please step out and share what you are feeling with those you love.

- Thirdly, allow people to visit. Even if you don't feel or look like yourself, the company is good for your mental health, and it keeps you in touch with the world.
- Finally, try to create a routine to focus on, as this breaks down your day into manageable chunks.
- If you are bedbound, try to keep your mind as occupied as possible. Read, watch films, listen to podcasts, do puzzles, write poems, draw, do anything that fills your time, as sometimes having too much time to think can play havoc with your mental health.

Today I am grateful for

DAY 2

Task

What have you become scared of? How can you fight the fear?

1 _____

I can fight it by

I can fight it by

Today I am grateful for

DAY 3

Dentist Helen Clint BDS (Hons), MJDF (RCS Eng)

All of this advice is general advice, based on current guidelines, so be sure to see your own dentist for specific treatment or individual advice.

What would you like pregnant women to be aware of regarding their dental health while pregnant?

Lots of changes happen to your body during pregnancy, but did you realise that pregnancy can also affect the oral health of some women? It can potentially put them at increased risk of tooth decay – this is largely attributable to changes in dietary patterns and gum disease, due to increased pregnancy hormones affecting your body's response to plaque. Your plaque control may be the same as usual but your body's response to dental plaque is usually more severe.

How can people protect their teeth in pregnancy?

Pregnancy does not automatically damage your teeth and the old wives' tale warning women to expect a tooth to be lost for every baby is not true – calcium is not taken from teeth in pregnancy. Dental issues are largely preventable, so with sufficient oral hygiene practices at home, and professional care from a dentist, you can keep your teeth healthy throughout pregnancy.

Bleeding gums, strange and sweet cravings, altered taste sensation, morning sickness (that can sometimes go on for the day and beyond the first trimester!), having a gag reflex when attempting to brush your teeth and changes in your dietary habits can all have a negative impact on your oral health. Naturally, growing a baby takes priority at this time, but being aware of your oral health in pregnancy is important too.

Clean your teeth thoroughly twice daily with an appropriate fluoridated toothpaste (this can prove difficult if you have a strong gag reflex as a result of pregnancy). Sometimes it may help to change the time of day that you clean your teeth and it may help to use a smaller toothbrush, such as a toddler toothbrush. Concentrate on your breathing during toothbrushing, and you could try using an alcohol-free mouthwash in the morning. Mouthwash can also be useful if you have morning sickness, as rinsing with this or plain water will help to prevent the acid in the vomit from attacking your teeth. Do not brush teeth straight away after vomiting as the enamel on your teeth may be softened by the acid in your vomit. Wait at least 30 minutes after being sick to brush, as this will allow the mouth to return to a more neutral state in this time. Sometimes milder-tasting toothpastes can help if the nausea is related to the flavour rather than brushing itself. A few episodes of vomiting are unlikely to cause any lasting damage; however, repeated vomiting (and/or reflux, i.e. regurgitating food or drink) can potentially damage tooth enamel.

Hormonal changes in pregnancy can make your gums more sensitive to plaque, leading to swollen (inflamed) and bleeding gums, which is known as pregnancy gingivitis. Occasionally, some women will develop a localised swelling on their gum known as a pregnancy epulis and this usually resolves after childbirth. It may be that there is a pre-existing gum problem that becomes more evident in pregnancy and this could be gum disease. Your dentist will be able to make an accurate diagnosis.

In the UK, dental care is free during pregnancy (currently with a valid maternity exemption card, so ask your doctor, nurse or midwife for form FW8) and for one year after your baby is born. When you go to the dentist, make sure you inform them that you are pregnant. I am often one of the first people that my patients will inform of their pregnancy but rest assured that we treat this information confidentially and will not discuss outside of the dental surgery.

Is there any dental treatment that people should not have while pregnant?

Dental treatment is generally safe during pregnancy, but some of your treatment options may be different when you are pregnant and your dentist may defer some treatments until after your baby is born, particularly in the late stages of pregnancy to avoid you lying back in the dental chair for a long period of time. Local anaesthetic (what we use to make you numb) is generally very safe – we use a relatively small amount and the most commonly used local anaesthetic is lignocaine (also known as lidocaine) which is fine to use throughout pregnancy.

You may wish to discuss with your dentist if any new or replacement fillings should be delayed until after your baby is born. The Department of Health advises that amalgam fillings should not be removed during pregnancy (if you are in pain, your dentist can discuss how this can be managed, for example by using a 'rubber dam' to isolate the tooth). Although there is no evidence that amalgam fillings are a health risk, these are not recommended during pregnancy or while you are breastfeeding. If you are in pain your dentist may stabilise your tooth and restore it more definitively postpartum. We would also advise deferring any cosmetic dental treatments until after pregnancy, as tooth whitening is not recommended during pregnancy or while breastfeeding. If you need a routine X-ray, your dentist will usually wait until after you have had the baby, although if one is absolutely necessary, the X-ray doesn't point towards your developing baby and is considered safe. However, your dentist will discuss this with you on an individual basis.

What other advice can you offer?

Prevention is always best so in general we encourage regular check-ups, so that your dentist can give targeted and individual preventative advice. It is one less thing to worry about throughout pregnancy if you know that you are dentally fit.

With regard to diet, if you are hungry in between meals, try to snack on fruits and vegetables and resist the urge for sweet treats. Try to avoid regular consumption of sugary and acidic foods. This might not always be possible during pregnancy, particularly if you have severe sickness and food aversions or cravings and are having to eat little and often. As I previously mentioned, having a healthy pregnancy takes priority, but when your sickness subsides, get back into a healthier regime. When you are pregnant you must have a healthy, balanced diet that has all the vitamins and minerals you and your baby need. Calcium is particularly important, to produce strong bones and healthy teeth. Calcium is found in milk, cheese and other dairy products. Cheese is also great for teeth as it returns the mouth to a more neutral environment.

Pregnancy is also an ideal time to quit smoking. Stopping smoking will reduce the risk of complications in pregnancy and birth and smoking is also one of the main causative factors in gum disease and oral cancers.

It's amazing to think that by eight weeks pregnant, the tooth buds of a baby's teeth are distinguishable and, by 20 weeks, the tooth buds of your baby's adult teeth start to develop.

Today I am grateful for

DAY 4

Support – Prenatal depression

I think prenatal depression is still an under-recognised condition (this is the term for depression that develops during pregnancy), and so many people suffer from it in silence. Just because someone has prenatal depression doesn't automatically mean they will suffer from postnatal depression, but it does make the person more at risk from it.

For this reason, if you are experiencing prenatal depression, I would advise having a support system in place for the period following the birth, so you limit the chance of feeling overwhelmed if the depression doesn't lift.

So why do people get prenatal depression?

For some, it may be due to hormones, for others it's brought on by battling troubling pregnancy symptoms. For others, it may be due to unresolved grief, PTSD or other mental health issues (possibly previously suffering from depression) or for many different reasons. The important thing is to get help, so you don't feel like you are suffering in silence. Getting good support can make all the difference.

Today I am grateful for

DAY 5

Journalling your pregnancy

What gestation is your baby today? _____

How big are they? _____

What symptoms are you now feeling?

What do you want to remember about how you are feeling or what you are experiencing?

Pregnancy post-loss can make you completely obsess about tiny, seemingly irrelevant things. This is your brain's way of trying to take back control, as nothing makes you feel as utterly powerless as grief and pregnancy.

ZOË CLARK-COATES

Today I am grateful for

DAY 6

Support – Fear of postnatal depression

I had the fear of postnatal depression (PND) during every pregnancy, yet I never had a trace of PND at all. Having gone through loss, I was genuinely concerned that any unprocessed grief and feelings might appear as PND. One well-meaning friend who had suffered from PND also felt the need to tell me I was at risk of it, and that made me feel like I was a ticking time bomb.

So firstly, just because someone you know has suffered from PND that doesn't mean you will. Likewise, just because you have gone through loss or trauma, that doesn't mean you will get PND.

So can you do anything to avoid it?

I don't think you can really, apart from ensuring you have a good network of support around you when you have your baby, but there are some things that may help:

- Keep talking about your feelings, fears and concerns and try not to internalise them.
- Don't feel you need to act like a superhero . . . everything shouldn't be your responsibility! There is an old saying that it takes a village to raise a child, and this is so apt. Accept help and share the load and responsibilities with others.
- Try to get as much rest as you can, as sleep deprivation can negatively affect mental health. If someone offers to come and babysit so you can have a daytime nap, say 'YES please'; grab every chance to sleep with two hands.
- Your home doesn't have to look perfect. When you have a newborn, you often have to choose to overlook the mess you are surrounded by. Try to look beyond the dust, the crumbs on the carpet and the pile of dirty laundry, and focus on this special time with your baby instead.

- Ensure you eat well, drink lots of water, and remember to take care of you as well as your family. Self-care isn't something anyone should feel guilty about; by looking after yourself you are benefiting your family long term.

If you do get any symptoms of PND, please avoid searching the internet for advice that may not be relevant to you, and instead talk with your doctor, midwife or health visitor. The support is there if you need it.

Today I am grateful for

DAY 7

Journal

If you could plan your perfect three meals in a day, what would they be?

1 _____

2 _____

3 _____

Have you gone off any food in pregnancy?

Have you gained any new food passions in pregnancy?

• •

Sometimes you need to just weep
on the floor and that is OK.

• • • • • • • • • • • • ZOË CLARK-COATES • • • • • • • • • • • • •

Today I am grateful for

WEEK 27

. . . .

DAY 1

Support – Panicking about your life changing

People often think it's bonkers to worry about their life changing when they have longed to have a baby, but let me reassure you that any concerns you have about this are completely natural. Worries are often just your brain's way of trying to process and come to terms with life radically changing. When you have no idea how things will look in a few months' time, it is normal to have the odd panic and concern.

So how does one address it? Write a list of all the things you are fretting about. Are they things that can be addressed or are they things only time will reveal? For example: concern over having less quality time to spend with your partner. Worry about having enough money when you are on maternity leave. Can these concerns be tackled head-on? If the answer is yes, think about doing just that. If they are things that you can't do anything about, try to talk about them with someone you trust, and try to find a sense of peace in the waiting.

Having a baby (or increasing the size of your family) involves colossal adjustment for you and your partner, and any other children you may be raising, and it's important to let yourself have time to adjust to changes that have happened or are due to happen.

The crucial thing is, please do not feel guilty for any anxiety you have. Being scared about how life will be after the birth of your baby in no way changes the love you have for your child, or your desire to be a parent.

Today I am grateful for

> [ ]

DAY 2

Task

Have you become pessimistic about life? Write down two areas where your thoughts have centred on the negative and then write down how you feel you could change the way you think.

1 _____

I can change this thought process by:

> [ ]

2 _____

I can change this thought process by:

> [ ]

Today I am grateful for

DAY 3

Esther's Story

Pregnancy has never been easy for me. My first pregnancy was a complete surprise, and I struggled to feel bonded to the baby growing inside of me. I had extreme morning sickness and spent the first four months in and out of the hospital. I waited for the glow to come, and it never did. I found pregnancy uncomfortable and exhausting. I watched other pregnant ladies enjoying newfound confidence in their bodies and a sense of glow, and all I felt was exhausted, sick and dull. My zest for life was drained from me, and I found my usually bubbly extrovert personality dulled and subdued. I had a great labour and birth with my first, and once I held my baby in my arms, to my utter surprise, I knew I wanted more children, but I was not prepared for what was to come.

I fell pregnant nine months after having my first. We were ecstatic, though I dreaded the pregnancy and sickness. Just weeks later, my world came crashing down as I experienced my first miscarriage. I went on to have two more miscarriages between each of my three subsequent children, each time being missed miscarriages. Emergency scans showed no heartbeats and I gave birth to my babies, born too soon, at home.

My last miscarriage was between my third and fourth full-term pregnancies, where I lost twins. I was rushed to hospital as I was losing so much blood and it was the most traumatic experience of my life. The medical staff and my husband were amazing, but I suffered PTSD and extreme anxiety afterwards and I have pretty much blocked out from memory my final pregnancy for my fourth child as I was so anxious and exhausted.

All of my full-term pregnancies were complicated, and this meant pregnancy for me was never easy. Pregnancy post-loss was mainly a test of endurance. It felt like a journey where I just had to survive for nine months. I was incredibly sick for the first four months. Often I would be sick without warning and remember finding bins, office drawers, bushes and other corners to be sick into at random moments of my day. At four months, I would usually start to feel extremely worn out and would have to take to my bed by mid-afternoon every day.

In my last three full-term pregnancies, by five months pregnant I had a diagnosis of obstetric cholestasis which is a liver disorder in pregnancy and gives intense itching. This meant daily blood tests and extra monitoring and taking medication to manage the symptoms. Looking back, I realise I just blanked most of my pregnancies out. I was emotionally exhausted from my previous losses and was obviously anxious, but at the time, I managed it by going to my bed and numbing all feelings and thoughts. I remember watching other pregnant ladies rubbing their tummies and realising I never did that. I felt bonded to my babies, but I was always wary of getting 'too attached' as I had previously, which meant I saw pregnancy as a route to a baby and nothing more. I didn't glow, and I certainly didn't enjoy it. I spent the last two to three months of each full-term pregnancy in bed almost continually. I had to be signed off work early, and my husband had to look after everything – children, work, household – while I lay in bed. I was so aware that so much was out of my control, that my babies had been taken from me and I couldn't stop it, that I went into myself and my safe place.

I cocooned myself physically and emotionally; during that time, I allowed my body and soul to just be still and to hibernate. I didn't process, and I didn't evaluate, and pregnancy was not something I cherished or feared, it was just nothing. For me, this was the way I protected myself but it was also how I healed. I gave myself rest, and I let myself be. I was lucky enough to have a support network and supportive husband to allow this to happen, but also I think I would've let everything drop anyway because I couldn't carry on. I hated being pregnant, and nothing would change that, but I knew I wanted to do it to have my precious baby. So I watched box sets for eight hours a day and lay in bed, only getting up for meals or to go to the toilet. I feel guilty now. So many ladies who loved being pregnant talked about the bonding time, taking baths to watch their babies kick – I couldn't do that and felt like something was wrong with me because I had such a negative and difficult experience of pregnancy. It put a huge strain on my marriage and my mental health. Thankfully I managed to have the right people around to support us and help us through, but it could've been so different.

For me, the butterfly moment of pregnancy was giving birth. My cocooned state would come alive as soon as I went into labour. I loved giving birth and had the privilege of having very easy and straightforward labours. The midwives joked that I loved labour so much because I knew it meant I wouldn't be pregnant anymore, but I think there is truth in that. I found I bonded with my babies during those short hours of labour more than in all my pregnancies combined.

My glow came during birth; people commented on how amazing I looked after labour. I felt like my hibernated soul had now awoken and was allowed to love and be loved, and I almost instantly got my energy and zest for life back.

Pregnancy for me was hard and horrid and a very difficult time of my life, but it gave me my babies, and for that, I am truly grateful. I still marvel at what my body did, that it carried eight babies, four to term and four for just weeks. But that doesn't mean I enjoyed it or even that it was OK. It was awful. It was excruciating, numbing and the most difficult times of my life. But I know that even the hardest of moments bring the most beautiful joy. I wanted to share my story to say that if you are struggling to be pregnant post-loss, or you find pregnancy difficult and resent it, it's OK. I did too. We all have a different story to share and not all of us glow on that journey.

Today I am grateful for

DAY 4

Support – Marking loss anniversaries when pregnant again

So many people struggle with loss anniversaries or other key dates surrounding the baby they lost, and they can feel this even more when pregnant with another child. Some people feel guilty publicly grieving while they are pregnant, as they worry it suggests they aren't grateful for the baby they are carrying. Let me start by reassuring you that of course this isn't the case, and anyone who suggests it to you is wrong. Grief and gratitude can and do run side by side. Feeling one emotion in no way means you don't feel the other.

The second concern people often have is that the baby they are carrying will feel rejection if they are grieving for another baby. Again, your baby will not be aware of your grief; they will just be aware of your love for them. Finally, people often worry that acknowledging a sad date or occasion will mean they spiral into a black hole of grief. I would kindly suggest that by not allowing yourself to process your feelings and sorrow, you are way more likely to encounter a grief wave when you least expect it. Let me, therefore, encourage you not to fear any dates, but instead see them as an opportunity to deal with another grief layer.

Today I am grateful for

DAY 5

Journalling your pregnancy

What gestation is your baby today? _____

How big are they? _____

What symptoms are you now feeling?

What do you want to remember about how you are feeling
or what you are experiencing?

. . . .

When you are pregnant post-loss
it can feel like you are trapped
in a world of
'what ifs'.

. . . . ZOË CLARK-COATES . . . .

Today I am grateful for

> [blank box]

DAY 6

Support – Health niggles

I don't know if anything prepares you for the enormous changes your body goes through when it is pregnant. You expect the backache, stretch marks, tiredness, but there are so many other medical niggles that can take you by surprise. There are far too many to list here, so I will mention a few I dealt with.

- Restless legs and arms – This is so rarely talked about and it affected me most nights and felt torturous. The only thing that brought me relief was Andy massaging my arms and legs.
- Hip pain – It hurt to walk but it also hurt to lie down. Two things helped me. The first was I purchased a thick memory-foam shower mat and laid it on the bed under my hips. Having this under me seemed to relieve a little of the pressure on my hips when I lay on my side. The second thing that helped me was sleeping with a pillow in between my knees. This kept my legs apart and made it more comfortable to sleep. Your midwife or doctor may refer you to a physio or another specialist if the pain is troubling you and they may be able to help relieve some of your symptoms.
- Nausea – When pregnant with Esmé I managed to control the symptoms enough with food and the majority

of the nausea passed at 14 weeks' gestation. The sickness and nausea with Brontë lasted throughout the pregnancy and I had to take medication to control the symptoms. Food that helped me included ice lollies (especially Mini Milk lollies), rich tea or arrowroot biscuits, citrus sweets (especially lime Starbursts), oven-baked potatoes, crackers with a little cheese. I found eating small amounts often was a lot better than eating full-size meals. Eating something before getting out of bed in the morning also helped. Please don't just suffer in silence if the nausea or vomiting is too much to bear, your doctor can help you.

- Piles/haemorrhoids – There is so much I could say about these but I will refrain, although trying to avoid constipation certainly helps . . . I didn't avoid it, thus why I could fill a book on the woes of suffering with piles! Regular warm baths can help if you are suffering, and speak to your doctor or pharmacist about good topical creams to apply.
- Indigestion – I often felt like I had a physical fire burning in my chest, and again I had to resort to medication as no natural solution helped. Speak to your doctor if you are suffering.
- Headaches – I suffered with headaches from the moment I found out I was pregnant up until my girls were in my arms. There are many things you can do to help the symptoms if you too are suffering. Take time to rest, as tiredness can make them worse. Avoid screen time as much as possible. Rest with a very cold flannel over your eyes and forehead. Ask your partner or a caring family member to rub your feet (this really helped me). Take time to properly relax and spend time in the outdoors, as carrying tension in your body can make headaches worse. The most important thing you need to do, however, is speak to your midwife and doctor about any headaches or migraines, as there can be underlying reasons for

suffering with them, so it's essential you tell the people who are looking after you.

I did feel like I was experiencing the A to Z list of pregnancy complaints, and I didn't want to complain about any of them, as I was so blooming grateful to be pregnant.

How many of you feel the same? It is so hard when you have wanted something so badly to then feel like you have no right to complain about anything to do with pregnancy. Let me reassure you, it is fine to complain, and if and when you do, it doesn't make you any less grateful for this baby you are carrying. You are human, and pregnancy is tough, and that's only talking about the physical side of pregnancy, not the emotional and mental battle you have to face. Once in a while, give yourself permission to have a whinge and share your health niggles with those who will understand and support you.

Today I am grateful for

DAY 7

Journal

How can you be kinder to yourself? List at least five ways.

What can you do that would benefit yourself five years from now?

When . . .

When . . . you find it hard to remember
the last time you looked
forward to something.

When . . . you don't remember
a time when you weren't
consumed with fear.

This is the time when you
need to hold on.

When . . . you need to trust
life will get easier.

When . . . you need to believe
happiness is on the horizon.

When . . . you need to trust that
tomorrow could possibly be 'when'.

ZOË CLARK-COATES

Today I am grateful for

WEEK 28

● ●

DAY 1

Support – Sleep deprivation

There is a reason sleep deprivation is used as a torture tool – only those deprived of it can adequately grasp the severity of the symptoms it can bring. Lacking sleep can make you feel ill, drained, confused, weak, emotional, and so much more. If you are struggling, please speak to your doctor as there is help available.

Exercise in the day can benefit sleep patterns at night, so if possible try to incorporate some physical movement into your days. My personal advice includes switching off all electronic devices an hour or so before you go to bed. Try reading or something else that relaxes you.

- Darken the room and dim all lights as you start to unwind, so your brain is getting prepared to switch off.
- Avoid caffeine and sugar from 1pm, as these can both cause sleep issues.
- Have a bath or a shower and use a relaxing scented body wash or bubble bath. Certain fragrances such as lavender, vanilla, sandalwood, juniper, lemon, bergamot and frankincense can alert your brain to sleep being imminent. I also like to use these fragrances in room atomisers or pillow sprays to scent my bedroom.

What if you fall asleep easily, but wake and can't get back to sleep?

My top five tips for going back to sleep are:

1. Switch on a mindfulness app or play audio books. Hearing someone quietly speaking can stop me mulling things over in my own head. I have this ready by my bed, just in case I wake up, so I can switch it on easily and stay in a half-awake, half-asleep state. If you prefer to listen to music add *Sleep* by Max Richter to your playlist. Max worked with neuroscientists to create this stunning piece of work. It has eight hours of music designed to help you sleep and rest.

2. Try not to look at the clock. Seeing the time will just make you end up doing sleep maths . . . i.e. *how much time do I have left in bed?* If you work out that you now have little time to get more rest, that can make you panic and this surge of adrenaline makes it even harder to get back to sleep.

3. Don't look at social media, emails or anything that makes you want to react. You want to encourage your brain to switch off, not reactivate.

4. Some people like to get up if they are really struggling to go back to sleep. For me this is a no-no, as then I know I will stay up. If it works for you though, try it. Keep the lights dim, and perhaps read something that encourages you to relax. Avoid starting physical activities, as it is vital that your body at least rests when you are pregnant, so, even if you aren't able to sleep, relax and let your body gain strength.

5. Drink something – If you have had a nightmare, drinking a glass of water can really help, as sometimes nightmares are caused due to dehydration. With this in mind always keep water by your bed, so you don't need to get up if you are thirsty.

Today I am grateful for

DAY 2

Task

What are the thoughts that haunt you? Write them down. Once these emotions are expressed or verbalised, they can at times dissipate, as they are often just seeking to be heard.

Today I am grateful for

DAY 3

Dr Jessica Farren MA, MBBS, MRCOG, PhD, OBGYN

As a doctor, what advice would you give to someone who is pregnant after a loss?

I think it is important to remind yourself that the odds are heavily stacked in your favour and that you are very likely to have a healthy and uncomplicated pregnancy.

I would also recommend reminding those around you, and any medical professionals you see, what you have been through, and explain why you may be more anxious than someone who has not been through loss.

More than anything, I think it is important to be kind to yourself and to accept however you feel, whenever you feel it. You may find it incredibly difficult to be excited about the pregnancy or feel unable to bond with the life that is growing. You may find yourself cautiously optimistic – but then berate yourself for 'tempting fate'. You may hate every minute of being pregnant and feel guilty about this. There is no right way to feel.

Sometimes, women will find that anxiety symptoms get significantly worse during a subsequent pregnancy after loss. Some women experience symptoms of post-traumatic stress disorder (PTSD) in a subsequent pregnancy, which may result in them having nightmares or flashbacks about their previous losses. Or they may struggle with reminders of previous events – going to the antenatal clinic, or the labour ward, are common triggers. If you have noticed any of these symptoms, then you should speak to your GP or hospital doctor and look to be referred for some specialist psychological support and/ or treatment. These sorts of symptoms can have a significant impact on your quality of life, and on your ability to enjoy motherhood, so they are important not to ignore.

I am suffering from PTSD following a loss. What advice can you offer?

The most important thing is to get help. You should speak to your GP about your symptoms and ask for them to refer you for treatment. The therapy recommended is usually cognitive behavioural therapy, also called CBT.

Today I am grateful for

```
┌─────────────────────────────────────────────────┐
│                                                 │
│                                                 │
│                                                 │
│                                                 │
└─────────────────────────────────────────────────┘
```

DAY 4

Support – Different pregnancies

Every pregnancy is different, so however much you want to compare this pregnancy to a previous one, you must accept it will not be the same. It is natural for your mind to try to evaluate a situation and try to collate all data in an attempt to bring you peace, but you have to try to remind yourself this is a new pregnancy and a new situation. Even if you have the same symptoms, the outcome is highly likely to be totally different this time.

I also want to address the feelings that arise when medical people, or friends and family, don't view the baby you have lost as just that – a baby. This can be so challenging emotionally and mentally. If people devalue your previous pregnancy due to an early gestation (or for any other reason), it can feel and seem like they are saying the baby who died didn't matter. Of course that will make most parents' blood boil. Before you know it, you are trying to defend your baby's worth and honour, and the whole focus of the discussion has been lost. If you have someone on your medical team who does this, or a family member, I would recommend telling them immediately how you feel. Tell them that however early or late your loss was, you lost a child and would like their existence to be acknowledged.

Today I am grateful for

DAY 5

Journalling your pregnancy

What gestation is your baby today? _____

How big are they? _____

What symptoms are you now feeling?

What do you want to remember about how you are feeling or what you are experiencing?

I have never known anything
as effective as grief at showing
you what truly matters in life.

It has a way of revealing the truth
and reinforcing the value of
the people around you.

ZOË CLARK-COATES

Today I am grateful for

DAY 6

Support – When your insides don't match the outside

It can be so hard to explain to others when everything on the outside looks fine, but inside you feel in pain. To the outside world, you may appear to be healthy and happy, and expecting a longed-for child. On the inside you may be filled with fear and anxiety. If you try to express this to others they may tell you to think about how lucky you are, which only makes you feel guilty.

You could be sitting at a perfect beach resort, looking at the most stunning view, and you still feel utterly crap. Whether this emotional turmoil is due to hormones, life events, grief, health or some other factor, it is tough to verbalise this kind of emotion when things seem fine on the outside.

If you can determine a reason for this sensation, I encourage you to work through those emotions to try to rebalance yourself.

If you can't get to the bottom of why you're feeling emotional, it can help to just think of it as something you have to ride out. Sometimes these feelings leave as quickly as they arrive, and you have to try to get through the duration of their visit as best you can.

Today I am grateful for

DAY 7

Journal

What gifts did your childhood bring you, and what do you hope to teach your child because of them?

. . . .

I don't want friends who just like to
sit with me in the good times.

I look for people who will come
searching for me if I am quiet.

Those who, if they find me in a hole,
will get a ladder and climb in to sit with me.

Real friends do life with you.
The good, the bad and the ugly.

. . . . ZOË CLARK-COATES . . . .

Today I am grateful for

WEEK 29

● ●

DAY 1

Support – When you no longer trust your own body

Trusting your own body can be a real challenge for people post-loss. During any subsequent pregnancy, you will be told hundreds of times to 'trust your body' (especially if you do a hypnobirthing or antenatal course), but what happens when you don't trust your body anymore? What happens when instead you blame your body for losing a baby in the past, and you no longer have that faith in yourself or your anatomy?

The first thing I would suggest is talking about your feelings surrounding your previous loss. This isn't a little thing to do, it's a big thing. For some, it may feel too huge to take on right now, and I get that, I really do. Talking is the key to uncoupling this belief system that your body is to blame, but if you choose not to do that right now, or it's merely not possible currently, how do you move forward?

I would suggest you practise some of the relaxation exercises in this book, and while doing them think of positive things about your body. Be thankful that your heart continues to beat. Your hands have the ability to write. The more gratitude you can feel for your body the better, as you want to try to replace negative thoughts with positive.

When negative or self-critical thoughts take hold, try to remind yourself that you and your body are not to blame for any loss. Unfortunately, we don't control how we're physically created, and we have no control over our genetic makeup, so even though people often carry internal guilt, it's mostly false guilt, and at some point this ideally needs to be addressed.

Try to practise empowering your mind and your body to

believe in itself again. Whatever has happened in the past, you need to try to trust your body, believe it will do the best it can in the situation it is presented with.

None of this is easy – it is probably one of the biggest battles you will encounter in pregnancy following a loss. Sometimes you need a group of people around you, cheering you on, encouraging you and reassuring you that your body can do this.

I believe in you . . . do you believe in yourself? If not, keep working at it, as you can change your thought patterns over time.

Today I am grateful for

DAY 2

Task

Write down exactly how you feel today, then pluck up the courage to tell someone else what you have written.

Today I am grateful for

DAY 3

Anna's Story

My first-born child, Erin, died when she was 22 days old. It had been a stressful and worrying pregnancy, and we knew that she might be born with health complications; however, we never expected she would die. Tragically Erin was born with a congenital heart defect, and despite surgery to try to save her life, she died in my arms before we even had the chance to take her home.

Following Erin's death, I could not imagine having another child. I didn't want another baby; I just wanted my baby; my darling, precious Erin. However, over time, the ache of being a mother without my baby to hold in my arms became too much, and just seven months after Erin died, I found out I was pregnant again.

Finding out I was pregnant came with a complex mix of emotions. I felt joy, but then guilt. I felt excitement, but then almost paralysing fear. I wanted this baby; a sibling for Erin, but I also desperately wanted Erin. It was difficult to navigate the rollercoaster of feelings. At the time of falling pregnant, I was still on sick leave from my work as a clinical psychologist following the death of Erin. I had received bereavement counselling – my first experience of being on the 'other side of therapy', and in many ways felt that I should be able to manage my feelings of anxiety and fear. After all, I spent my working life listening to, supporting and helping others manage their worries and difficulties. So for many months, I tried to struggle on alone. I don't think anyone apart from my husband knew how terrifying this pregnancy was for me. Our friends and family were so happy for us – they had witnessed our grief and devastation at Erin's death, and I know they wished us future joy. However, I was terrified that this pregnancy was in some way erasing Erin's memory and that a new baby would make others forget her. I feared that others would think our new baby was replacing Erin and this fear brought with it immense feelings of guilt and shame. I worried about how I could possibly be a good mother to both Erin and her younger sibling. It felt as though I was in an impossible situation. If I felt joy for the new baby, I felt I was betraying Erin, but if I didn't feel the joy, I felt as though I was letting down my unborn child. I didn't know how to cope with and manage these conflicting feelings and my mental health suffered.

Also, I felt overwhelming fear that this baby was also going to die. I spent every day of the pregnancy wondering if this would be the day I would hear those awful words, 'I'm sorry, there is no heartbeat.' It wasn't a case of worrying if the baby would die; there was no if in my mind. I lived every day of that pregnancy certain that I was not going to take a living baby home. This was my experience, and my fear did not allow me to look outside of that. However, if I dared share these thoughts with the many health professionals I saw throughout the pregnancy, they did little to help me. I lost count of the times I was told, 'this time will be different', 'this baby is healthy' or 'all will be fine this time'. These statements did not help. In fact, they made me feel more alone and isolated because I did not feel as though anyone was listening to me. The result was that over time I stopped sharing my fears and I was left to suffer alone. I felt heavily burdened by the responsibility I felt to keep this baby alive. In my mind, I had let Erin down, and in my vulnerable emotional state, I thought it inevitable that I would also fail this baby.

Somehow I struggled through to around 34 weeks. I was back at work and functioning OK there, distracting myself and trying not to think about the pregnancy. I became an expert at putting on a cheerful face and speaking light-heartedly about the baby. However, deep inside, my fear was at an all-time high. I couldn't bear to attend antenatal classes and bought essentials needed for the baby with reluctance and trepidation. I did attend a hypnobirthing class in the hope it would help with some of my anxieties, but I left halfway through in tears. I felt out of place among the happy and optimistic pregnant ladies who made up the rest of the class, and I was terrified about the prospect of being asked if this baby was my first. What answer could I possibly give? It would destroy me to deny Erin's existence, but how could I talk about my baby who died to these joyful, carefree pregnant women? It felt cruel and wrong, and so I left, crying all the way home as I felt more and more alone.

It was around this time that my husband insisted I reach out for help, and so I contacted the bereavement nurse at the hospital. I now know this is something I should have done much sooner. She helped me immeasurably. It wasn't that she could take away my fear, but she listened to me and didn't try to dismiss it. So although the fear remained, I was no longer feeling alone with it. She arranged for me to speak to midwives about the birth so that it could be planned as much as possible, which brought me some comfort. She also arranged for me to have regular monitoring at the hospital so that I could hear the baby's heartbeat and feel reassured that, for that day at least, the baby hadn't died.

Due to my fears and fragile mental health, my baby was induced at 38 weeks. I remained terrified, although the midwives were very kind and empathic towards me. Unfortunately, the induction process did not progress – I believe I was just too scared – and so my son was born by C-section. He was beautiful, and more importantly, completely healthy. The fears and certainty I had held for the past eight months that my baby would die turned out to be completely false. Furthermore, my heart was bursting with love for him and this love did not take away any of the love or grief that I held for Erin. I was now a mother to two babies, one I would hold forever in my heart, and one who I was lucky enough to also hold in my arms.

I have now had two further children; Erin has two younger brothers and one younger sister. All the pregnancies have been difficult and full of fear, and my heart will forever grieve for Erin. The birth of her siblings has not taken away any of the pain at her loss. However, they have brought more joy, laughter and hope to my life. My three younger children are growing up knowing all about their brave big sister, and now I know that I can be a good mother to all four of my children and should be able to do this without feeling guilty. For as long as I live, I will talk about and love Erin so she will never be forgotten, the birth of her siblings cannot change that.

Today I am grateful for

DAY 4

Support – Establish aftercare support

Once you get your baby in your arms, you will need time to process and adjust following this long mental battle you have been through. Of course, at that point, you will also be taking care of a baby who is entirely dependent on you, and it is easy to forget what you have walked through for the past nine months (possibly way longer if you had recently lost before conceiving again). That is why you must put a care plan in place for yourself – right now! No, you really shouldn't wait until your baby arrives, as at that point all focus will be on him or her, so you ideally need to do it NOW.

Do you have anyone you can trust who will agree to come and sit with the baby a few times a week? If you do, book them now. Then plan to use that time to sleep, rest, meditate, bathe, etc. This time shouldn't be used to do laundry or other household chores; this time is your time. It is about giving yourself space to process what you have been through. Time to think and process further layers of grief. Time to re-engage with the feeling of peace, which may have seemed elusive for quite some time. I promise you this will be the most significant gift to you and your baby, and you will be so thankful you arranged it before your little one's arrival.

Today I am grateful for

DAY 5

Journalling your pregnancy

What gestation is your baby today? _____

How big are they? _____

What symptoms are you now feeling?

What do you want to remember about how you are feeling or what you are experiencing?

Some people have a natural ability to make
others feel rubbish about themselves.

You have to decide whether you allow this or not,
as no one can make you feel bad without your permission.

So set your boundary lines high and wait
for your happiness levels to soar.

ZOË CLARK-COATES

Today I am grateful for

DAY 6

Support – Fear of the world

A fear of all the bad things that are happening in the world
is so natural when you are pregnant or post-birth. I would
often wonder how I hadn't noticed before that the world was
so full of unbelievable disaster possibilities. Wars, terrorism,
murders, pandemics, you name it, I seemed to hear about it
all when pregnant, and every bit of news scared me. Here
I was bringing an innocent baby into the world, and it felt
like there was evil on every street corner. So how do people
handle it? For some the best way is to avoid listening to the
news: you may need to create a safe bubble for yourself if it's
seriously troubling you. You won't be able to screen out all
the news, but even if you can avoid half of it, you may feel
less overwhelmed.

Secondly, you need to search out good news – look out for

stories about good people, awe-inspiring people, people who are making this world a better place.

Finally, practise interrupting any negative thoughts that are circling in your brain. Tell yourself that more good happens in the world than bad. There is way more chance that the future will be good rather than catastrophic. Try to stop yourself from spiralling into a negative thought pattern, which can easily happen if you have an active imagination. Remember that you are not your thoughts – sometimes we have to try to take charge of our less helpful thoughts and rein them in.

Today I am grateful for

DAY 7

Journal

What is the most difficult emotion for you to experience, and why?

Which three qualities would you like to nurture in your personality? For example, I would love to become more patient, as I find it so hard to wait for news, and this impatience increases my stress levels.

1 _____

2 _____

3 _____

. . . .

People are often quick to envy others
for a life they have,
but what if they only have a
happy life due to the rocky
path they have walked?
What if they only have children
following years of tragic loss?
What if they only experience so
much joy because they grabbed hold
of happiness with both hands,
following years of harrowing pain?
Would others still envy the
life they now lead?
Perhaps the grass is only greener
as it has been watered with tears.

. . . . ZOË CLARK-COATES . . . .

Today I am grateful for

WEEK 30

DAY 1

Support – Superstition

When the bottom has previously fallen from your world, I think it's natural to want to try to prevent further disaster, and that's when fears and superstitions become a common reaction. You may feel like you might jinx things if you don't act a certain way.

I often hear people say, 'I can't have any baby equipment in my house until after the baby is born, as it's bad luck to have it before.' Or, 'I have to wear the same outfit to every scan, to ensure I only hear good news.'

I personally don't believe in superstition; I happily walk under ladders. I don't mind how many birds I see outside my window, and I never 'touch wood'. For me personally, these are old wives' tales and hold no power. I worry that a lot of superstitions risk making people feel responsible for accidents and adversity, and likewise make them scared of future doom, should they inadvertently cross a black cat. But for some, superstitions are a big part of their life, and they can even help people feel more in control. If, however, you feel controlled by superstitions and rituals, and want to feel freedom from them, try to identify what you are fearing and where the fear originates from. Just by addressing your worries and concerns you may feel less inclined to conform to superstitious rules.

Today I am grateful for

DAY 2

Task

Use these spaces to write down any misconceptions you feel people have surrounding your loss. Then do the same for those around your current pregnancy.

How do these make you feel?

Today I am grateful for

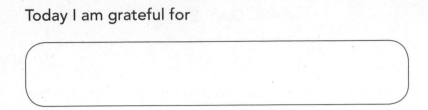

DAY 3

Clare Bourne MCSP, MHCPC, MPOGP, Pelvic Health Physiotherapist

How do I prevent vaginal tears during birth?

Most women approaching birth understandably fear vaginal tears. A high number of women will have an element of tearing, but this doesn't mean the tear will be big. The best thing to do running up to the birth to prepare and prevent tears is perineal massage, and there is good evidence to support its use to reduce the risk of tearing or need for an episiotomy.

How do you stop abdominal separation occurring during pregnancy?

Lots of women are concerned about abdominal separation, known as diastasis recti. This is where the distance between the six-pack muscles (rectus abdominis) gradually widens, and there is stretching of the linea abla, which is the connective tissue that joins the muscles together. Unfortunately, we can't prevent it, and studies have shown it is present in 100 per cent of women by the end of pregnancy, so be reassured it is a normal part of pregnancy that needs to happen to allow your baby to grow. You can help look after your tummy muscles during pregnancy by rolling over onto your side to get out of bed and generally avoiding movements that cause a bulging or tenting down the middle of your tummy. There is a natural improvement in these muscles after birth. If you feel you are having ongoing issues with your tummy, please do seek medical advice and request a referral to women's health physiotherapy. It is understandable to be worried about exercise and movement after birth if you feel you have a separation, but exercise can actually really help, and movement is the key to recovery.

For all of the topics mentioned, there is help at hand, and women's health or pelvic health physiotherapists are widely available. We are here to help and want to stand with women during this time in their lives.

Today I am grateful for

DAY 4

Support – Breastfeeding or bottle?

Believe me, this is something I didn't even know whether to include in these pages, as I didn't want a storm of controversy around the book.

So all I will say is this.

You do what feels right for you and your baby. No guilt. No pressure. END OF STORY.

I see so many people suffering from depression and guilt as their feeding didn't go to plan. I want you to enjoy being a parent with as little remorse as possible – so whether you breastfeed or bottle-feed, I hope it makes you and your baby healthy and happy.

PS: I didn't have one single drop of colostrum or milk come in with any of my pregnancies – none, zilch! I don't think this makes me a freak of nature (please don't message me if it does; I prefer living in denial). So I chose bottle-feeding, or bottle-feeding perhaps chose me, and I loved it. My husband and I both got to feed our daughters, and it was such a special time for us as a couple. I never felt any guilt or worry about this, as my daughters were flourishing on the milk we gave them. I hate to think of any mum feeling bad for any choice they make on this. Just relax and be confident with the decision you make, or your body makes.

Today I am grateful for

DAY 5

Journalling your pregnancy

What gestation is your baby today? _____

How big are they? _____

What symptoms are you now feeling?

What do you want to remember about how you are feeling or what you are experiencing?

Today when you criticise yourself
for not being happy enough, for not being chatty enough,
stop and remember the heartache you have endured.

Instead of condemnation, feel pride.
Pride that you are still standing.
Pride that the grief that could have destroyed you
has actually made you a more compassionate,
more caring and kinder human.
Pride that even when you were terrified,
you had the courage to try again.

ZOË CLARK-COATES

Today I am grateful for

DAY 6

Support – Do babies run out of room at the end of pregnancy?

No, they don't. So if your baby's movements change at all – increase or decrease – from what you're used to, call your midwife. This old wives' tale has caused countless issues over the years, and we need to dispel it fast. Your baby should have a typical pattern of movement, and this shouldn't alter at any point in your pregnancy, however big or small your baby is – so don't fear speaking up if you are worried. Call your midwife. Call the hospital. If you don't get a response go to the hospital. Nine times out of ten, you will be given complete reassurance that your baby is totally fine, but that shouldn't stop you from calling the following day if you have a similar worry. The only thing that matters here is the safety of your baby and you having peace of mind.

Today I am grateful for

DAY 7

Journal

Forgiveness is a powerful thing, and I have found that if I don't forgive people, I am the one who suffers, as the feelings and resentment gnaw away at me. Is there anyone you need to forgive? To forgive doesn't mean you are saying what they did was OK, or was acceptable, it just means, 'I am choosing not to live with this bitterness hanging over my head, so I make a choice to forgive and just focus on positivity moving forward.'

* *

When we lost our baby we didn't know
the language to use to explain the pain, the heartbreak,
the utter agony we were experiencing.

Over time we found some words
that aptly verbalised the grief, but what we learnt was
that there are simply no words to describe baby loss;
it goes beyond the vocabulary available to us all.

The same applies to pregnancy post-loss;
it is impossible to express the dichotomy
of fear and joy rolled into one.

To understand it, one must
have experienced it.

* * * * * * * * * * * * ZOË CLARK-COATES * * * * * * * * * * * * *

Today I am grateful for

WEEK 31

DAY 1

Support – Emotional resilience

Often we have no clue where our resilience and strength may come from – we can feel both weak and strong in the same day. Hope and fear, dread and excitement, peace and terror – all swing in and out of focus, often with no warning. Sometimes situations alter our emotions, but at times a feeling can dominate our thoughts for no apparent reason.

How is it that we felt peaceful yesterday, but today we're racked with torment and worry? Who knows – our brains are confusing organs, and the fact that no one has a mind remotely the same as anyone else's means we will probably never understand our own thinking, let alone another person's. Perhaps we should all therefore reluctantly accept that it's OK to feel it all, and agree that it doesn't need to make sense to us or anyone else – we can deal with whatever feeling is currently holding the most prominent space.

It is wise, though, when our emotions are all over the place, to pay attention to how well we are looking after ourselves. It is a lot easier to feel emotionally stable if we are prioritising rest, relaxation and eating well.

Today I am grateful for

DAY 2

Task

Do you have a mantra? A mantra is a positive sentence that one repeats regularly, either in the mind or out loud. The words should focus your mind and motivate you to achieve something or overcome something. My personal mantra through pregnancy was:

I can do this, I will do this and my story will end well.

If you don't already have a mantra, why not create one? Write it on a piece of paper and stick it up in a place of prominence. Whenever you need to encourage yourself, seek it out and read it aloud. Let those words permeate your soul.

Today I am grateful for

DAY 3

Tyne's Story

Gravida: 5
Para: 0

This was the sad code at the top of my maternity notes that I made the mistake of googling. Five pregnancies and no live births, bleak reading, even if this time I had made it far enough along to have maternity notes.

Our baby journey began shortly after getting married. With tans still fresh from our honeymoon, I had an early miscarriage. Barely days after seeing that second line on the test, I'd started to bleed. We took it on the chin, no one knew except our very closest people. I didn't have to talk to anyone. The pregnancy had inspired us to look at our life and buy a bigger home and I thought this was really positive that we had learnt something from this 'test'. We got healthier, started taking vitamins and focused on starting married life with our 'bad luck' behind us. I reasoned I was only 30, my mum had had a miscarriage shortly after getting married, and she went on to have five healthy children naturally, not even having drugs in labour. Confidence renewed, bodies and minds strong, we decided to try again.

A year later . . . In what will surely (?!) be the worst year of my life, we, in very quick succession, had three ectopic pregnancies in 10 months. I'd never even met anyone who had experienced one ectopic pregnancy, let alone three!

The three enormous blows shattered what optimism I could muster. Ectopics, I learnt, were a whole different ball game – conversations about internal bleeding, two emergency surgeries and the third treated with a type of chemotherapy. My husband Dan had faced the very real possibility that I may not be OK as my tube ruptured and I was raced away from him in blinding pain.

The surgeries meant I had enforced time off work to recover, so everyone quickly knew what had happened. My employer was incredibly supportive, never putting pressure on me to come straight back to work. I, however, chose to carry on as much as possible; but with each loss, my resolve was harder to summon. I became angry; I drank more; I became quite lost. I'd wait the three months that I was recommended, and then we would try again. But despite the confidence of my consultant and no reason or risk factors against me, luck was never on our side.

After 10 months, I was left with a broken soul, physical scars, and one sad fallopian tube that had been so traumatised that doctors didn't know if it would work in the future. I was never going to have a baby naturally now. I felt so vulnerable, so exposed and so very empty. The NHS offered counselling; I went along to a sad therapy hut in Slough and dutifully sat with the stranger and mumbled away but what I needed was my husband. He was as much a part of this as me. We found the more we talked, the more it helped, and we became so close and united in our grief. I am fortunate he is a more open person than me, less prone to tears and naturally more optimistic and vocal about his feelings. We bumbled through each day, waiting for the next stage of our story.

Luckily in my area and with my age and circumstances, I qualified for IVF. The postcode lottery with fertility funding is famously hit and miss, but I was so grateful for the glimmer of hope this offered. The waiting game continued, as referrals slowly led to appointments, injections and finally the wait to see if a second line appears on the test and if *this time* baby is in the right place.

The first embryo transfer we did worked, and we saw that blessed second line for the fifth time and began the worst of the waits – seven weeks for the 'viability scan', where they check the location of the pregnancy and if there is a heartbeat.

Throwing up from nerves on the day of the scan and so jittery I couldn't drive, we immediately saw something we had never seen up to this point – the tiny circle in the womb and a flicker of a heartbeat! Faces wet with tears, we couldn't believe it. BABY IS IN THE RIGHT PLACE! Now we just had the small matter of the next 33 weeks to get through . . .

The pregnancy progressed, but still, I couldn't quite let myself give in to the excitement. Each week I took bump photos, always saving them to a separate folder on my phone . . . just in case. For weeks I panicked about bleeding, rushing to the loo multiple times each day to check. I don't think the anxiety and trauma of loss ever leave you. But little by little it did progress; I grew out of clothes and plans had to be made.

Outwardly I was cautiously optimistic; I said the right things to friends and family, but internally I was still a stone. I was barely daring to breathe. My past experiences were making me hard and afraid. My brain was keeping part of me protected from further trauma.

I did everything I was supposed to; I did the classes, I asked friends for advice, I made lists. Slowly, by 30 weeks or so, I'd bought the essentials. By 35 weeks I'd collected what I was being given by friends. In truth I was just going through the motions. Inside I was worrying, what if this didn't happen? What if the birth went badly? I could barely even think about it. I'd still physically catch my breath and gasp in panic sometimes.

I resisted my husband doing up the spare bedroom for the baby. It was fine. It had woodchip wallpaper and threadbare carpet, just as the rest of the house was as we moved in, but it didn't matter – if the baby arrived safely, he or she would be in with us anyway.

Stubbornly . . . in continued panic, everything I'd collected stayed in the spare bedroom in bags. My mum eventually intervened, she asked to come and stay with us, just her. She lives over an hour away, and family meetups are typically large, noisy and booze-filled occasions. She just wanted a 'moment' alone with me as she called it. Just us! This doesn't happen. She put the wind up me to get properly sorted. She is practical, not silly, full of love and gut Mother Earth intuition with what to do. She instilled in me what I had to do in the house and reasoned with my anxious, paranoid brain that all would be fine. We spent time looking at the tiny clothes I'd bought and washing and organising it all. I slowly started to unwind. Little by little my brain unknotted.

I got round to reading a book I'd been given on birth. I was engaging finally with the pregnancy. The book's purpose is to dispel negativity and empower women to trust in their bodies and be clued up with birth choices and the process of labour. It was easy to read and funny. For the first time, I felt that I could do this; one more major milestone to pass, and this baby would be with us. The conception may have been artificial, but the birth would be all me. My resolve was strengthened. Anxiety had turned to determination, and I gritted my teeth and faced the last stage – the birth.

Finally, before I'd started my maternity leave, at 38

weeks my waters broke. This was real. Painfully real. From 1am to 6am my body – achingly slowly – got to 2cm dilated. TENS machine nearly at maximum and my meditative state weakening, I opted begrudgingly and in desperation for pethidine, other pain reliefs and the labour ward only being available to women over 4cm. Then in the blink of a (drowsy) eye, I was pushing, and an hour after that her head was born, and this tiny little face screamed up at me before the body was even born! One final big push and she was here, flopped onto my chest, covered in gunk, all squished up but blooming perfect 6lb 15oz of real-life healthy baby. My baby! She has her daddy's nose and red hair and is vocal, sassy, funny and confident.

We called her Pia Hope, after my mother.

We finally did it; she was here! All of the losses, the tears, the waiting, the injections, the dark days were suddenly over. Pia Hope, you are everything we ever wanted, thank you for making me your mummy xx

Today I am grateful for

DAY 4

Support – Fearing blood loss in labour or delivery

If you have post-loss fear around blood, the idea of blood loss in labour or delivery can be a huge issue. I always encourage people to talk with their midwife about this, as they can quickly and easily reassure you of what to expect and tell you what is normal, so you don't freak out.

I never saw any blood loss with my daughters as I had two C-sections but I still worried that one day I would go to the loo and lose my plug, so I understand this worry.

For many people blood is a massive grief and panic trigger post-baby loss. It can even continue each month when a person has their normal cycle. So how do you stop it being a trigger? You can probably guess what I am going to say – yes, counselling. Ideally, a course of CBT would be beneficial.

If you don't manage to stop the trigger before having your baby, please don't overly worry, you will be absolutely fine. If you feel upset or panicked, the medical staff should be able to reassure you quickly. Additionally, try to take time each day to practise relaxation exercises, as the more you do them, the better you will become at being able to relax in stressful situations.

Today I am grateful for

DAY 5

Journalling your pregnancy

What gestation is your baby today? _____

How big are they? _____

What symptoms are you now feeling?

What do you want to remember about how you are feeling
or what you are experiencing?

· ·

You know when it hurts like hell to
talk and explain how you feel?
Well, that is exactly when you
should share your feelings.

Pain can only start to heal
when it is expressed.

Fear can only be overcome
when it is faced.

· · · · · · · · · · · · ZOË CLARK-COATES · · · · · · · · · · · ·

Today I am grateful for

> ┌─────────────────────────────────────┐
> │   │
> │   │
> │   │
> └─────────────────────────────────────┘

DAY 6

Support – Fear of having a newborn

Just because you have longed for this day doesn't mean you don't have the right to fear it, struggle with it or feel under pressure to enjoy it. The fact that you have wanted this for so long truly can make the prospect of a newborn baby even more daunting. Likewise, you can feel genuinely unprepared for bringing home a baby. When you haven't even dared consider that you may have a healthy child to raise, and your only focus has been on getting through pregnancy and keeping your child alive, when you do suddenly make it across the finish line it can be a real shock!

So how does a person deal with this?

- You allow yourself to feel it all, and admit to feeling it all.
- You confide in someone who will understand (if you don't have someone, find me out and tell me), as airing those fears diminishes their power, and you can then (I hope) start looking forward to having your little one in your arms.
- Don't be embarrassed to tell your family and friends your worries either, and if you can share your concerns with someone who has a small baby themselves, even better. Ask them if you can spend the day with them, watching and helping. You will quickly discover all

parents develop their own childcare patterns, and you will do the same when your little one arrives.

My best tips for preparing practically for a newborn are:

- Have a large quantity of nappies ready. If you are using disposable nappies, buy a few different brands to try out, as we found the size and shape of your baby can make a big difference when it comes to which brand to purchase. Some nappies always leaked on us, so we had to keep switching makes.
- Have all baby clothes pre-washed and ready in a drawer. I couldn't believe how many sleep suits we went through in that first month. I think Esmé had to be changed around five times a day, as she would always dribble milk. Babies grow out of the tiny newborn clothes so fast, so I would not spend too much money on the very tiny outfits; spend your pennies on clothes from three months upwards. Clothes with press-studs are easier than buttons.
- You can never have too many bibs and muslin cloths to drape over your baby when feeding and winding.
- Decide whether you want to offer your baby a dummy/ pacifier/soother. Esmé refused to have one, while Brontë loved hers.
- If you are feeding with formula, stick with one brand. Only change if the milk isn't suiting your baby. We gave all milk at room temperature as the hospital told us it was much easier, and I am so glad we did, as it meant we could feed the girls anywhere.
- The girls both had mild colic – Infacol really helped them.
- The best piece of equipment we ever bought was definitely a baby carrier – both of the girls were super-happy in this at all times!

- Best toy? Esmé never depended on a toy to help her sleep, but Brontë loved her bear that played white noise. Yes, it is incredibly annoying for adults to hear the sound, but it really helped Brontë settle in her cot, so it became one of those vital toys we never dared be without.
- Nappy/changing bags – Always keep one stocked, so you can grab it night or day and know it has everything you need in it. Have at least one complete spare outfit in it at all times, including a spare coat (we learnt this the hard way on multiple occasions!).
- My other top tip is, if you have a car, keep a spare emergency outfit for you in it. You never know when your baby may deposit some type of fluid on you. The amount of times I would require a change of outfit when out was staggering.
- If your baby cries when you change their nappy, try draping a muslin cloth over their chest and stomach, as they often cry because they hate the feeling of the air touching their skin.
- Babies' vests are designed to be removed either way . . . over their feet (so downwards) or over their heads (so upwards); it's why they have extended neck holes and slits in the material. I only found this out when my children were older – if you didn't know this, you will thank me for telling you one day!

These are some of the things I wish I had been told.

Today I am grateful for

DAY 7

Journal

What were your favourite storybooks as a child? Compile a list and try to find copies of these to pass on to your child.

My friend, today may be hard.
Today may feel overwhelming.
You may wish you could just hide under
the covers and will the day to go away.
But let me reassure you:
You can survive it. You will survive it.
Take it a minute at a time.
Before you know it another 24
hours will have passed.

ZOË CLARK-COATES

Today I am grateful for

WEEK 32

● ●

DAY 1

Support – Fear of cot death

This was a real worry for me, not only because I knew all about this subject, but also because I had a well-intentioned but worry-inducing health visitor who made it her mission to instil the fear of cot death – or sudden infant death syndrome (SIDS) – into all new mums.

So how do we cope with facing this subject, especially when we want to avoid it from ever happening?

I found the best way to look at it was from a scientific angle. I looked at the stats and the data. I read that as long as I followed all the latest advice, my baby would be as safe as they could be and that when people followed all this advice, the risk of incidents was tiny. Yes, I know we all want the threat to them to be zero, but that can't happen here, so we have to limit as much of the risk as possible, and then trust all will be well.

We used baby monitors with sleep pad alarms (which were both good and bad for us, as when we had them falsely go off, boy did they increase the fear!). We didn't have any bumpers in the cots or loose blankets or toys; plus, we followed all the rules when it came to sleeping positions.

I do not include safe sleep advice here, as the guidelines change so regularly. I would prefer you to get the latest leaflet and information from your midwife or health visitor when your baby is born.

This is one of the times it sucks being a parent. You want guarantees. You want to know for certain that your baby will be OK at all times. But, sadly, you can't always know that, and by navigating this fear, by doing all you can to keep your little one safe, and then learning to relax and trust they will be OK, you are practising a vital skill that will be useful to you for the whole of your child's life.

Today I am grateful for

DAY 2

Task

Write down your current worries and fears

Most people's worries originate in the thought of what *could* happen, rather than being due to what *is* happening. So I'd like you to write two separate lists, the first being a list of things you are worried about that are actually the case right now, and the second a list of things you are worried may happen in the future. It can be helpful to see these written in black and white, as that in itself can help reduce some of the panic one may be feeling.

Things I am worried about that are currently the case

> Things I am worried about that haven't happened

Today I am grateful for

DAY 3

Dr Jacque Gerrard MBE, Midwife Consultant and former Director for England at the Royal College of Midwives

Are you able to choose which way to give birth? Including requesting a C-section?

Yes. It is important that women are offered choices for all parts of the maternity pathway, including place of birth, pain relief, infant feeding choices and pregnancy screening, etc. Women can request a C-section which, in general, is safe; however, there are risks associated with this. It is therefore important that the woman has a detailed discussion with an obstetrician and her midwife, and hears the evidence about risks associated with a C-section so that she can then make a truly informed decision about her birth mode.

Why do people say babies move less towards the end of a pregnancy? And what happens if every day you are worried about baby movement?

This is a myth. Babies move throughout the pregnancy.

It is important that women are aware of the baby moving and the pattern of movements throughout the pregnancy. If a woman feels that her baby's pattern of movements has changed in any way, it is crucial that she contacts her midwife or doctor to get a check-up. All women in England are given an information and advice leaflet at the latest by 24 weeks gestation explaining the importance of foetal movements and patterns. This advice is discussed with the woman at every antenatal visit and contact with the midwife. This is part of the safer maternity care bundle.

Never sit and worry, call your midwife.

Today I am grateful for

DAY 4

Support – Your truth matters

If people don't acknowledge your loss, it doesn't mean it's not important. If those around you ignore your pain, your worries, your fear, it doesn't mean it's not significant.

If loved ones or friends don't rally to support you, it doesn't mean you aren't worthy.

Don't let others define you or your experiences.

- You matter!
- Your story matters!
- Your struggle matters.
- Your truth matters.

So confidently speak about what you are feeling and find those who will sit and listen to you sharing your heart.

Today I am grateful for

DAY 5

Journalling your pregnancy

What gestation is your baby today? _____

How big are they? _____

What symptoms are you now feeling?

What do you want to remember about how you are feeling or what you are experiencing?

Don't tell me to just be grateful for the children I have. The moment you utter those words, you are telling me I don't appreciate my children, which is the worst insult of all, as they are my world. Secondly, you are minimising my loss. Being grateful will never negate the pain and grief of losing a baby.

ZOË CLARK-COATES

Today I am grateful for

DAY 6

Support – Shame

Shame is one heck of a powerful feeling. It has the power to hold us hostage. So what has shame got to do with grief and loss and pregnancy after loss? Sadly, a lot. It is very common for people to feel huge levels of shame surrounding their baby loss. People often worry that they may have been responsible for their baby dying, which means they feel shame discussing their grief. They feel shame about how they processed their grief, or perhaps how they didn't progress through grief as they felt they should. An example of why people carry shame in pregnancy following loss is feeling dreadful that they aren't able to celebrate the pregnancy, since they are so fearful that their baby will die. This can bring about feelings of shame as they know so many others never get the chance to carry another baby post-loss.

The issue with shame is it often tries to silence people. It can be very difficult to open up about your worries if you fear you may be judged for them. It can also be hard to verbalise the outcomes you may secretly fear.

Can I encourage you to speak up, to share with someone you trust all the areas you feel burdened with shame, as just by talking, you can find freedom! By allowing yourself to engage in a rational conversation, the lies and confusion that shame brings to the table can be seen as just that – lies and things that are simply not true. Once shame is lifted, you will find you are able to talk about your experiences and losses, and journey with more ease.

Today I am grateful for

> [blank rounded text box]

DAY 7

Journal

Do you feel shame?

List areas of your life where you feel shame. If you feel responsibility or guilt, can you learn to forgive yourself? If, when you rationally look at these things, you can see you are not responsible for them, how can you free yourself from carrying false shame?

> [blank rounded text box]

Some of you are reading this wondering
how you can continue on.

I get it, I have pondered similar
thoughts in the past.

The weight, which right now feels
so utterly overwhelming,
won't necessarily become lighter,
but you, my beautiful friend,
will become stronger, and more
skilled at carrying it.

So hold on, even though you feel so weak,
you are in fact gaining strength.

ZOË CLARK-COATES

Today I am grateful for

WEEK 33

DAY 1

Support – Taking each moment as it comes

You don't have to have it all together, and you certainly don't need to feel every emotion all at once. Some days you may feel happy. Sometimes you may feel devastated. Some mornings you may feel hopeless, yet some evenings you may feel full of optimism. Every single day will bring new feelings and fresh challenges. You may wake up and see mountains before you, and you may fall asleep in the valley; this is the hard part of life – we have ever-changing scenery around us. If one can learn to embrace the new and the unknown, while simultaneously releasing things one desperately wants to hold on to, life can become more manageable. When the situation feels bleak, remember that the scenery will change – nothing is permanent.

Today I am grateful for

DAY 2

Task

What is the best advice you have ever been given?

What do you think the best advice you have ever given to someone was?

Are you following this advice? If not, consider how you can from this point forward.

Today I am grateful for

DAY 3

Laura's Story

Pregnancy after loss is hard. And yet, even typing that sentence, I feel guilty. Shouldn't I be grateful? Joyful? Of course, I am! 'The Fear' doesn't take away from how much I want to celebrate this little life inside me, but it does mean that I'm more cautious than I once was, less inclined to let myself look ahead too far.

This is pregnancy number four, in less than two years. Four beautiful babies who have known love from the minute I knew they existed. That in itself is amazing; two years ago I couldn't conceive, and we were waiting for IVF. Of course, that means that after each loss people would say, 'At least you can get pregnant now' as if that was the consolation prize. It's not.

We hoped this time, after some tests, that doctors would tell us why I kept encountering loss. Instead, we were told, 'There's nothing wrong, it's just one of those things.' I desperately hoped that there was a problem that they could fix with one small pill or one lifestyle change. Instead, I'm second-guessing everything I do: 'Is this bag too heavy?', 'Can I eat this?', 'Did I do this last time?' All the while, deep down, knowing that whatever I do, it won't change the outcome. So, I've swapped wine for folic acid, and we're waiting it out.

Loss takes its toll. This time around, when that second line appeared, all I could think was, 'Here we go again.' I feel so guilty about writing that. Like I wasn't happy or grateful. Of course, I was, so very grateful. But oh, so scared! I texted my family and close friends; this time, I couldn't face the rollercoaster of emotions that comes with telling them face to face or on the phone. I told them, 'I'm too scared to feel anything else right now, but you can be hopeful for us.' And they are, they have been ever since I told them I didn't know if we could conceive naturally.

But, I feel guilty. Like I haven't celebrated this baby in the same way. But that doesn't change my love for them. It doesn't change how wanted they are and how hopeful I am that we'll get to bring this baby home. I'm just constantly terrified.

Loss changes your language too. At some point, 'when' becomes 'if'. 'If I get to the first scan', 'if the next scan goes well', 'if I get to 12 weeks'. Ah, 12 weeks. That magic, hopeful number, I've never reached that point yet; as I write this I'm just over six weeks, I have seen my baby and their beautiful flickering heartbeat and now I'm waiting for another scan in two weeks, hopeful that we'll see them again: healthy, thriving, growing.

And I cringe away from 'congratulations' or 'you must be so excited for your scan'. Those words feel alien in among the worry and anxiety when it's taking all of me not to take myself off to bed for the next six or so weeks and wait it out.

When I tell people our news now (and I do tell people because I need support if the worst happens), I announce it in an almost blasé way: 'I'm pregnant, again, at the moment.' It's very much, *This is how it is right now, but I'm expecting that to change at any moment.*

All the while, well-meaning people are telling me 'just think positive', 'a positive attitude helps'. No, it makes no difference. If a positive attitude had kept my babies alive, I'd be holding them today. A week or so into this pregnancy a friend of mine prayed with me; she said something so freeing: 'God, help Laura to realise that her mindset doesn't change the outcome of this pregnancy.' I was so grateful; although I knew deep down that was true, it was so good to be reminded of that and to have some guilt alleviated.

Time changes too. Whereas before I was counting week-by-week, checking my app to see what fruit my baby resembled this week (raspberry was my favourite, but I'm still holding out for pineapple: if you're immersed in the infertility world, you'll probably know why!). Once you've experienced loss, you start counting day-by-day, sometimes hour-by-hour, often toilet trip by toilet trip. You are obsessively checking that you haven't started bleeding, questioning every twinge. Each morning I wake up and thank God that I've made it through to another day with this baby.

Then their comparison. Passing milestones: 'By this point in my last two pregnancies I'd already been to the hospital', 'By this point I'd already lost a baby', 'No bleeding by this point is a good sign.'

And yet, this time, things feel different. This is the first time I can visualise this pregnancy progressing. There are times when I can see the pregnancy announcement, see my bump in a maternity dress at my sister's April wedding, see my May baby in my arms. But, as soon as I let myself go there, I chastise myself for getting ahead. I can't change it, though, and as a good friend once told me, you can't prepare for the bad news.

So we wait, and we pray. We let others love and support us. We tentatively talk about the future. We let ourselves feel how we need to feel. We let our dog distract us. And we hope.

Update: Since writing this piece Laura's baby made it safely into the world, and she now has a lovely little boy.

Today I am grateful for

>

DAY 4

Support – When to prepare the nursery

There is no right or wrong time in terms of gestation to decorate the nursery or buy baby equipment; the only right time is when you are ready. Some people choose not to decorate a bedroom until their baby is in their arms and at home, and I completely understand this. As the baby is likely to be sleeping in your room for the first six months, you have plenty of time to do this. I decided I wanted to decorate a bedroom before my daughter was born; for me, it was part of preparing emotionally for her arrival. I loved sitting in her room while stroking my pregnancy bump, imagining life with her in that space. Every time I sewed something for her room or folded a blanket in her chest of drawers, I took a step closer to the belief that I would bring her home.

When we delay physically preparing for a baby, I feel we risk not preparing emotionally for bringing a baby home. Raising a child (especially raising a child after loss) takes an enormous amount of energy, both emotionally and physically, and the nine months of pregnancy is not only about growing a child, it's also about transforming into that child's parent emotionally. So yes, preparing a room or space in your home may feel daunting, but if you feel able I encourage you to do this, as I think the rewards outweigh the emotional risk.

Today I am grateful for

DAY 5

Journalling your pregnancy

What gestation is your baby today? _____

How big are they? _____

What symptoms are you now feeling?

What do you want to remember about how you are feeling, or what you are experiencing?

Telling yourself you are silly or stupid for
feeling fear or worry won't ever banish it; in fact,
it is more likely to haunt you.
Trying to prevent yourself from feeling any emotion
is a proven way to increase the issue.
The only effective way to navigate the feelings you are
battling is to acknowledge they are there, accept that past
trauma or life experience birthed them, and then try
not to give them a seat at your table, even though
you are aware that they are in the room.

ZOË CLARK-COATES

Today I am grateful for

DAY 6

Support – Coping with tiredness

Dealing with tiredness is a huge issue for most pregnant people. I wish I could assure you that the tiredness leaves once your little one is in your arms, but I would be lying. I often wonder if the tiredness one feels in pregnancy is a way of preparing a person for life with a newborn, but why do people struggle with it and how can one cope with it?

- If you feel tiredness is an issue, I would always suggest talking to your midwife or doctor, especially if the tiredness or exhaustion has come on suddenly. At times there can be a treatable medical reason why a mum-to-be feels tired and help or medication could be needed.

- If, after seeking advice, you know your tiredness is purely due to being pregnant I would suggest considering the following: remember you are currently doing something so mind-blowing it is hard to comprehend – you are growing an actual person in your body. No wonder you are tired; you are not only needing to keep your body going, but you are also having to keep two people going – this takes energy!

- Also remember that processing grief is always exhausting, so doing this while simultaneously pregnant is, of course, going to drain you of a lot of energy.

- And be aware that the constant vigilance of fighting fear can deplete anyone's energy reserve! Again this doesn't even take into consideration someone being pregnant while facing daily worry and panic.

It is also worth considering that most pregnant people struggle with sleep, so they may not be getting the amount of rest they physically need to feel energised. Women say that their sleep is often reduced due to the need to visit the loo countless times each night, and they struggle with being able to get comfortable in bed. But there may be other things that you could tweak which could help. Try not looking at your phone or other devices for an hour or two before you go to sleep. Try to avoid drinks with caffeine after lunchtime, as they can act as a diuretic and increase the need for regular loo visits. Try to use cotton bedding and wear 100 per cent cotton clothing to sleep in as that helps your body regulate temperature better than wearing synthetics. Finally, try to practise your relaxation exercises each night before you go to sleep.

The reality for most pregnant people is that they will experience some level of tiredness at points, or throughout their entire pregnancy, and you must be kind to yourself if you experience this. Try to reduce your daily work commitments if possible and schedule a time each day to relax and unwind. Accept offers of help if they are made, and don't be afraid to ask for help if you feel you need it. There are no awards for doing everything on your own, so treat yourself like you would treat a friend, and make rest and relaxation a priority throughout your pregnancy.

Today I am grateful for

DAY 7

Journal

What are some of your helpful and unhelpful habits? What can you do to increase the habits that support you and let go of those that don't?

Because you feel they experienced a worse trauma doesn't in any way devalue yours.

Because the world says another loss was more significant than yours doesn't make that a correct fact.

The truth is your pain is not in competition with anyone else.

Trauma and loss are not something to be ranked or graded; they're relative to each and every person.

So allow your pain to be heard, to be appreciated and acknowledged.

ZOË CLARK-COATES

Today I am grateful for

WEEK 34

DAY 1

Support – Language surrounding loss

Time and time again in interviews, I'm asked to explain how I feel about 'having unsuccessful pregnancies'. I appreciate that those interviewing me are just struggling to phrase questions appropriately, but I would like to gently suggest that saying my babies who died were 'unsuccessful pregnancies' is not the best way to phrase this. I'm aware that if this is said to me all the time, it's probably told to many of you also.

I struggle to explain why it's so offensive to me, but let me have a go . . .

My babies were firstly not just a pregnancy. They were (and are) my children. Secondly, they weren't unsuccessful; they died. Would someone term a three-year-old who died 'unsuccessful' because they didn't live until they were four? No, of course they wouldn't, as the length of a life doesn't determine its success or value or worth.

So I suggest that we all gently correct those who use poor language, as we may be able to stop the world describing these precious children who died as unsuccessful pregnancies.

Today I am grateful for

DAY 2

Task

List five friends or family members who make you feel emotionally stronger. What do they do to help you achieve this?

1 _____

2 _____

3 _____

4 _____

5 _____

Notes:

Today I am grateful for

DAY 3

Dr Jessica Farren MA, MBBS, MRCOG, PhD, OBGYN

Why does loss happen?

The majority of early losses (approximately seven out of 10 early miscarriages) are due to genetic abnormalities, which means that the body has recognised that it is a pregnancy that cannot form a healthy baby. When the egg meets the sperm, an incredibly complicated set of reactions needs to take place to assemble the right amount and configuration of genetic material – and, when one of these misfires, sadly there is nothing that can be done to reverse that change, or for a healthy baby to result. In these situations, there is nothing that you can do, or that medicine can do, to change the outcome. A miscarriage may be the result of bacterial or viral infections in the mother, even when there are no symptoms of infection.

Sometimes miscarriage can be caused by problems in the way the blood clots, which may affect how the pregnancy receives its blood supply. Conditions such as antiphospholipid syndrome can be effectively treated by blood-thinning medication.

Losses caused by delivery of the baby before it can survive outside the womb

Sometimes this is associated with infection, including bladder infections, and at others it may be caused by a weakness in the cervix (the neck of the womb), which may result from previous surgery.

Occasionally, a baby passes away inside the womb. If this happens after 24 weeks of pregnancy, it is known as a stillbirth (as opposed to a miscarriage, which is before 24 weeks in the UK). It may result from a knot in the umbilical cord which supplies blood to the baby, or from the placenta not supplying the baby with the nutrients it needs to grow and survive.

There is still a lot we don't know about the causes of miscarriage and stillbirth, and we aren't always able to find a cause. Thankfully, there is lots of research taking place to understand better why losses happen, and to try to prevent them.

Why are people so often told there is no reason for their loss?

I don't think anyone should ever be told there is 'no reason' for their loss – only that the reason has not been found.

In early losses, this is mainly because genetic issues cause the majority of losses, and these are not routinely tested for: it is simply assumed that this is the problem.

In later losses, even if a woman or couple agrees to have every investigation offered to them (including a postmortem), in one out of two cases the cause cannot be found. This undoubtedly reflects our inadequate understanding of why miscarriage happens, and the inadequate ways we currently have of testing for problems. Hopefully, in years to come, we will be able to give much more satisfactory answers.

Importantly, if the message you have received is that there was no reason found for a loss, then there is nothing that you can or should be doing differently this time around.

Today I am grateful for

DAY 4

Support – Facing pain

Facing your pain is easy to say and very hard to do. When people look back on their lives, they often say it's the things that they did to avoid facing grief and pain that caused them the most issues. It's amazing how far we will travel out of our way to avoid dealing with trauma. The brain can make a person think that dealing with the pain is the same as going through it all over again, and that is simply not true. Of course, it is emotionally challenging and upsetting to process heartache, but by doing so, you move into a much better place, and it is worth shedding those healing tears.

Take some time to look back at your life. Can you see times when you have made certain decisions purely to avoid facing conflict or dealing with trauma? With the benefit of hindsight, do you believe those choices were the right ones? I believe we all get to a point in our lives where we have to choose to take the hard roads, even if we would prefer to go down the much faster slip road – perhaps this is part of maturing as an adult? I would wholeheartedly encourage you to choose to face your pain head-on, to not run from it, as I can promise you, life is so much richer when we embrace both joy and pain.

Today I am grateful for

DAY 5

Journalling your pregnancy

What gestation is your baby today? _____

How big are they? _____

What symptoms are you now feeling?

What do you want to remember about how you are feeling or what you are experiencing?

The important thing for you to
remember is you matter.

Your pain matters.

Your voice matters.

Your story matters.

Don't let anyone make you believe
otherwise, my friend.

ZOË CLARK-COATES

Today I am grateful for

DAY 6

Support – Relationships

Grief changes relationships not only with other people but also with oneself. I have witnessed confident people turn into insecure and emotionally vulnerable individuals overnight following a loss. As someone who works in the field this doesn't surprise me, but for many it can be confusing and upsetting to see how loss changes a loved one's personality or behaviour. I advise people to think of grief as physical trauma. I believe loss can leave huge emotional scars on the brain. People expect following an accident that any injured parties need time to rehabilitate. They understand that the injured person may or may not return to a similar version of themselves, but many don't offer the same grace to emotionally wounded people. I completely understand why this is hard – if one day you are happily going through life with your joy-filled best friend, and the next day they appear to be a completely different person, that's tough! Someone who is grieving may not even want to be around you – or anyone – anymore, and that can make friends experience feelings of grief themselves, as they mourn the friendship they once had. The result is a lot of hurting people who, while doing the best they can, may be unintentionally causing one another more pain.

So what can we do if we find ourselves in this situation? I would suggest being as real as possible about how one is feeling. We can't expect people to 'just know' what we are thinking, or what our needs might be. I would also suggest trying to empathetically look at everyone's point of view. It's easy to only look at one side, but by looking at how every party feels, your eyes can be opened to hidden pain being carried by people.

Today I am grateful for

DAY 7

Journal

Who do you admire and why? Pick someone who you respect for bravely sharing their story. What is it about their story that has increased your admiration for them?

. . . .

Fear is like a person hiding in the shadows,
but just a little light aimed in their direction
is enough to make them flee.

. . . . ZOË CLARK-COATES . . . .

Today I am grateful for

WEEK 35

● ●

DAY 1

Support – Considering our use of language

I am changing the language I use. I am going to stop saying, 'I am so sorry to hear that' when someone tells me of their sad news. I don't know why it's only just dawned on me that this is not the best language to use. I mean, I work in the field of grief support, surely it should have hit me before now? But hands up, I admit it, it only recently did so.

When we say, 'I am sorry to hear that', we aren't offering support, we are saying we regret hearing bad news. Now don't get me wrong, I know what the sentiment behind these words is: we are trying to convey our regret and sympathy. We are trying to say, 'We are so sad for you.' But 'I am so sorry to hear that' doesn't actually say that. Instead the phrase implies that hearing the bad news has been upsetting for us as the receiver in some way; as if we might prefer to only hear good news from our friends. Of course that is not what is intended, but words are powerful and we should all consider carefully how we use them.

Perhaps singular statements on their own have little power, but when we add them to the constant pressure levied against us all in society to hide our pain, I think they have an impact. Subtle messages to stay silent reinforce that internal voice, which is often very loud in our heads, that we should cry in private and just pretend to be happy for the sake of those around us.

I've resolved that, from now on, the phrase I will use instead is: 'Thank you so much for trusting me with your story. I am so sorry you are going through this pain.'

Let's all look at the words that we use, especially the

standard 'sympathy' phrases that we may say without much thought, and intentionally change the dialogue to be more encouraging and supportive.

Today I am grateful for

DAY 2

Task

What language could you change to help your emotional health or to help society become a better place?

Today I am grateful for

DAY 3

Bex's Story

Robbed. Robbed of the joy of it all. Those are the exact words I feel when I look back and remember my pregnancies, or when pregnancy comes up in conversation with friends.

We experienced three consecutive losses within the space of 18 months. Distraught, pessimistic and weary, we decided to give it one last shot after being given the 'all clear' by our wonderful consultant.

There were no jumping-for-joy selfies, phone calls or Amazon wish lists for us when we saw the positive pregnancy test one cold January morning. Just a few tears and a silent cuddle, knowing the potential heartbreak that might ensue. Looking back, this makes me so sad. There was no initial celebration for our child.

Fast-forward nine months to 1am on a September night, and our beautiful baby girl was being placed into my arms, healthy and oh-so-beautiful. If only I had seen that moment on that January morning.

But my optimistic nature had been crushed, and I had entered into my fourth pregnancy fearing the worst again. For the worst had happened and the worst could happen, and the worst did happen to us. Maybe there was a tiny bit of me that thought, 'This time might be different', and maybe that's what kept me going for those nine months. Perhaps I did have that glimmer of hope, but I never let it rise.

I had imagined, hoped, dreamt, fantasised, danced, shared the news with loved ones and shopped for baby paraphernalia before, and the hurt was too much when all that was obliterated in a moment. So this time I was going to do it all differently. There would be no 'looking forward' or daydreaming. I didn't buy a baby developmental bible – that meant getting too involved and attached. There would be no clothes shopping and no telling anyone. I couldn't bear the thought of letting them all down – again. And there would absolutely definitely NOT be a social media announcement. In fact, I never announced any of my pregnancies on social media.

I wish I didn't think like that. My family told me not to worry – 'It'll be fine.' Their reassurances went right over me as, the last time they told me this, it wasn't fine, it wasn't all OK, I lost my baby. I didn't need to hear general and easy reassurances, I needed to hear they understood how scared I was. They needed to recognise why I came across as off-the-scale paranoid, and why I just couldn't 'relax' and 'enjoy it'.

I was like this for my subsequent successful pregnancies too. Even when people told me, 'You know you work now, you can relax', it did not calm my paranoid, manic and anxious mind!

Our consultant told us that as soon as we found out we were pregnant, we were to book an appointment to see him so he could discuss medication options. This reassurance that we had a professional walking with us from day one was invaluable. But making that phone call to book an appointment was hard, really hard. I feared that I would have to phone them up later to cancel, explaining I no longer needed it as I was miscarrying. I had done this three times before, and it was agony. I also delayed making an appointment with the GP for the same reason.

We saw the consultant that week, and he prescribed a

progesterone pessary and aspirin. It felt good knowing I had a pharmaceutical boost to this pregnancy!

As the pregnancy progressed, and the bump grew, I would continually prod the baby to make it move, have a feel of my boobs to see if they were still sore (a good sign in my book) and take a quick trip to the loo to have a 'wipe' to check for blood. I must have looked a right sight (and reading it back now, it was crazy) but I didn't care. I needed constant reassurance. It took over my everything – my thoughts, my conversation, my Google searching – the need for reassurance that all was OK with my baby. I looked forward to every midwife appointment – they would give me the reassurance I craved, and I could listen to a healthy heartbeat. This 'peace' lasted 20 minutes and then I needed, wanted, craved more. It was almost an addiction, an obsession.

The fear crept into most of life's activities. I remember a holiday at Center Parcs, where I refused to ride a bike, swim for too long or eat certain things. I couldn't 'risk it'. We didn't ever go abroad while pregnant, and when we holidayed in this country, my husband made sure we booked somewhere close to a hospital. Man, that need for reassurance and security (for me, a hospital) was all-consuming.

On top of this, every trip to the toilet was excruciating. I became obsessed about checking for blood. It wasn't just me who had these unfounded fears. My poor husband used to dread phone calls from me (as this was how he found out about the previous losses) and watch with anxiety when I entered the room after yet another toilet trip: what is her expression – relief or utter pain?

Pregnancy after loss is hard, so hard. It is emotionally exhausting. No one told me that, and I didn't expect it. I carried my babies with anxiety, fear and pessimism.

I wish I hadn't, I wish I had had freedom, joy and optimism. If I did it again, I would work hard at accepting that whatever happens is out of my control and try to enjoy what is happening now. To enjoy the moment and to stop with the 'what ifs'. It makes me sad knowing I carried my babies with such negative feelings inside.

How sad that I didn't bond with my baby until I had her in my arms. I didn't want to get too attached, too involved. How sad that I didn't embrace the beauty of a pregnancy, how sad that I didn't engage with every single stage of growth, that I didn't laugh at all the quirks and peculiarities pregnancy brings, that I wasn't in awe at what my body was doing. How sad that I just wanted it over with quickly rather than appreciating the most miraculous, awe-inspiring event known to mankind and how sad that I just didn't enjoy the most precious and privileged nine months I will ever be gifted with.

I'm telling you this to encourage you to try to engage at every stage with your pregnancy. I didn't, and I missed out. I missed out on so much. My little girl deserved all of me during her time in my womb – my joy, my happiness, my celebration and my hopes for her. I understand completely how the fear paralyses you, the paranoia overwhelms you, and the pessimism overshadows you. But if somehow amid the fear, you can find a way to embrace this special season, it will ultimately bring you more peace. If you end up having a healthy newborn baby, you will be so glad you embraced that season of pregnancy and bonded with your baby. Even if the worst happens and you experience loss, you will know you gave your unborn baby your all, and that will be a comfort in the darkness.

Today I am grateful for

DAY 4

Support – Inability to feel excited

One of the significant changes I noticed in myself post-loss was I often failed to get as excited when good things happened, and it took me a long time to understand why. At first, I thought I was being overly cautious, holding back a little, just in case I was faced with more disappointment and heartbreak – and yes, perhaps there was a touch of this. I later discovered the main reason I wasn't able to feel excitement was that the physical sensation of excitement is very similar to the feeling you get when you are terrified. Your stomach flips, you get butterflies, and you can feel adrenaline pumping around your body. When you have an over-exaggerated fight-or-flight response due to experiencing loss, anything that triggers those sensations makes you panic. As a result, your brain learns to dampen all those emotions – so something that you would have previously been extremely excited about, you may now take with a pinch of salt. This may not seem like a big issue for some, but for me, it was a considerable loss. I am a very excitable person, and this change in me was something I truly missed. I am happy to say the feelings of excitement did return, but it took quite some time.

So how is this relevant to pregnancy after loss? Many people worry that they don't feel as excited as they would have hoped about their pregnancy. They fear that people around them will think this baby isn't wanted when that couldn't be further from the truth. I want to reassure you that if you are feeling this, please do not panic. Over time your mind will allow you to feel excited about things again, but for now, it's just trying to safeguard your emotions.

Today I am grateful for

DAY 5

Journalling your pregnancy

What gestation is your baby today? _____

How big are they? _____

What symptoms are you now feeling?

What do you want to remember about how you are feeling or what you are experiencing?

To the one who is struggling.

To the one who hoped it was just a bad day, but it turned into a terrible season.

To the one who is so scared to admit it hurts like hell, as they fear when saying the words they will simply break.

We see you.

We hear you.

We are standing right next to you in case you fall.

ZOË CLARK-COATES

Today I am grateful for

DAY 6

Support – Comparison with other pregnant people

Everyone's pregnancy journey is so different, but it can be super-hard not to compare paths with other pregnant people. We ask ourselves – why do they love the experience of pregnancy more than I do? Why are they not suffering from ailments as much? Why are they not scared of death? There are so many comparisons one can make, and questions one can ask, but comparison helps no one. All it does is make you feel anger, resentment, confusion and even guilt, shame and sadness. And yet comparison is so understandable, and it's often very hard to stop ourselves.

There is so much in life that doesn't make sense. Why is it not possible for some people to have children when they would make amazing parents, while others are having babies they don't want? Why are children dying of hunger, when others have so much food they throw it in the bin? There are so many scenarios that make us say, 'It just isn't fair' and, 'It doesn't make sense.' I think a turning point for me was when I finally accepted that life isn't fair. Not everything makes sense and I had to accept most questions I have will never get answered. My battle to find out why, and to make things make sense, was a big part of the reason I couldn't find peace. When I finally gave up doing that, and accepted the not-knowing, I was rewarded with new levels of contentment. I was finally able to accept that not every jigsaw piece fits into my final picture. That was a massive step forward in my bid to find peace.

Today I am grateful for

DAY 7

Journal

What do you want your family and friends to know you are feeling right now?

What do you want the world to know you are feeling right now?

It takes unbelievable quantities of energy
to try to appear fine when you
are so very far from fine.

ZOË CLARK-COATES

Today I am grateful for

WEEK 36

DAY 1

Support – Navigating grief

Navigating grief while trying to embrace life is a massive challenge, and I believe the secret to doing this well is facing the pain head-on. It means admitting what loss and grief have stolen from you, and then learning to develop new skills to journey through life.

I suggest writing a letter to your grief, to really confront those feelings we often prefer to avoid. What would you want to say to the grief you currently carry? See if writing it down helps the burden you carry feel less heavy. (This is the task for Day 2.)

Here is my own letter to grief:

Dear Grief,

I often refer to you as a gentle giant, an unwelcome visitor that society needs to embrace, as love brought you knocking at our doors.

You taught me so much . . . and brought me some treasured gifts. Because of you I am more compassionate, more empathetic and I truly embrace life.

But Grief, there is another side to you, a dark side, that I want to address.

Grief, you stole part of me, and it hurts like hell that I will never get that back. You crept in like a thief in the night and stole not only precious people who I love, but also the fearlessness that I had previously carried, and an optimism that was gifted to me at birth. You pulled the lever on a trap door that was hidden beneath my feet and, in the blink of an eye, everything was different.

This trap door, once opened, can never be shut. Once seen, it can never be unseen. Life now becomes about navigating the gap and doing one's best not to fall.

Those who we love, we fear we will lose.

Those who appear healthy, we dread becoming sick.

Life is no longer straightforward, simple or innocent. Life is now scary, complex, and a maze.

I want to tell you this, Grief, those parts of me you seized and robbed, I will weep for them for all of my days.

Zoë x

Today I am grateful for

DAY 2

Task

Write a letter to your grief.

Today I am grateful for

DAY 3

Dr Jessica Farren MA, MBBS, MRCOG, PhD, OBGYN

Can I request an early induction due to fear of going to full term?

Yes, you can. The doctor will, of course, want to explore your reasons for doing so and explain the process fully so that you understand the benefits and the downsides. Induction is generally very safe, and, after 37 weeks, does not seem to be associated with a higher chance of Caesarean section – but it is a different, and usually much longer (and so more tiring), journey to natural labour. The induction will take place in the hospital, and labour will be managed on the labour ward (rather than the birth centre), with continuous monitoring of the baby's heartbeat. Women with previous difficult experiences may find this reassuring.

If you previously suffered a loss late in pregnancy, the option of an early induction, or a Caesarean section, is usually discussed with you, as most women would find it difficult to manage the anxiety around the time of a previous late loss.

Can I request a C-section?

Yes, you can. However, your doctors will want to understand the reasons behind the request and will want to help you weigh up the risks and benefits of a Caesarean.

You may wish to have a Caesarean because you are afraid of labour itself – the pain or unpredictability – or because you will be able to feel more in control, knowing when you will have your baby, and how long it will take.

Probably the most important thing to consider about a Caesarean section is its implications for future pregnancies.

This may, of course, not be an issue for you. But repeated Caesareans are more likely to be complicated operations, with scar tissue, and a risk of causing damage to the organs that sit around the womb (the bladder and bowel). There is also a very slightly increased risk of a loss late in a subsequent pregnancy, for reasons that are not fully understood.

A Caesarean also usually takes longer to recover from than a vaginal delivery, and has some risks to your health – including the risk of blood clots in the legs and on the lungs, and wound infection. Babies born by Caesarean section may also be more likely to have some temporary breathing difficulties, and have asthma in childhood, or become overweight. Overall these risks are small.

It is for these reasons that, in a straightforward pregnancy, women are generally recommended to aim for a vaginal delivery. There are, of course, reasons why a Caesarean section may be recommended to you for medical reasons, for example if you have a low-lying placenta.

If you do choose to have an elective Caesarean section, it is important to remember that there is always a chance you will go into labour before your planned delivery date. In these situations, especially if the labour is advanced, it may be safer to continue with a vaginal delivery.

Today I am grateful for

DAY 4

Support – Losing your sense of self

Both loss and pregnancy, and even motherhood, can make a person lose the sense of who they once were. The person staring back at them in the mirror may no longer be someone they recognise. For some, these feelings are tolerable and just part of the journey of parenthood, but for others, they can feel overwhelming and scary. I think the less secure people feel in themselves, the more likely it is they will feel this way, especially if their self-worth rests on their abilities, rather than on who they are as a person. For example, if my confidence and self-assurance came from being promoted to director of a law firm last year, my self-esteem could plummet if, due to loss, I had to step away from my career. This is why it is so important to have your self-worth based on who you are, rather than on what you look like, do, or on what you own.

What can you do if you don't recognise the person in the mirror? I suggest you start on a journey to discover the new you. Work hard to find out what makes you happy, what brings you peace and, on the flip side to that, what makes you unhappy and makes you anxious. Perhaps you can do this through counselling, through journalling or just through talking through your feelings with your partner or a friend. Life is about self-discovery, and no one stays exactly the same. New beginnings and new starts can lead to new passions and hobbies. So if you feel that you no longer know who you are, choose to start finding out right now.

Today I am grateful for

DAY 5

Journalling your pregnancy

What gestation is your baby today? _____

How big are they? _____

What symptoms are you now feeling?

What do you want to remember about how you are feeling or what you are experiencing?

Most of the time we berate ourselves
for how we are doing,
but you know what?
We should be applauding ourselves
for navigating so much crap.

ZOË CLARK-COATES

Today I am grateful for

DAY 6

Support – Being kind to yourself

Why do we often treat ourselves in a way we would never treat our friends? Why do we push ourselves right to the edge of what we can cope with? Perhaps it's because we don't feel we deserve kindness and grace? Maybe it's because we were raised not to take time to heal, and we're encouraged to believe that never stopping is a display of strength? Whatever the reason, we need to apologise to ourselves and learn that our personal needs matter. We deserve to treat ourselves with compassion. Our pain, our grief and our wounds deserve to be seen and recognised. If you were to write a letter of kindness and forgiveness to yourself, what would it look like? It can be hard to think of how to address ourselves with compassion and understanding, so here is an example to get you started.

Dear Me,

Please forgive that I never gave you time to process the shock of the loss, and rushed you to recover. I apologise that I forced you to paint a fake smile on your face and pretend to the world that all was well, while your heart was silently breaking. I'm sorry that when your pulse was pounding, and your body shaking, I made you return to life, as I bought into the lie that I should appear like I was moving on, and my wounds were healed.

I hate that this resulted in you needing to hide in public toilets, weep in the car, have panic attacks in shops . . . You needed time, and I robbed you of that. I understand and regret that by me insisting on fake happiness, you wept endless tears in the shower, and those around you were unaware that you needed someone to dry your eyes.

Your loss, your pain, your heart cries. All of it deserved to be heard; I am genuinely sorry.

Today I am grateful for

DAY 7

Journal

What parenting skills did you witness as a child that you would like to implement when raising your own child?

. . . .

You can be both happy and broken,
optimistic and scared,
all at the same time, my friends.

. . . . ZOË CLARK-COATES . . . .

Today I am grateful for

WEEK 37

• •

DAY 1

Support – Anticipating delivery day

It is very hard to plan for something you have so little control over. If you are having a scheduled C-section, it may be a little easier to visualise and plan for the birth of your little one, but if you have a natural delivery, it's less easy. Either way, the wait to hold your baby may already feel like an eternity, and you may or may not feel anxious about the birth. For the purpose of this support section, I am going to presume you are nervous (or even terrified). If you aren't anxious about the birth, I am thrilled for you, and you may wish to skip this section.

Let me start by saying I entirely understand your fears. Most people who have encountered loss are constantly waiting for the bottom to fall from their world, and when you are not able to personally control the outcome of a situation, it can bring back all the old fears you may have battled with. So how do you cope mentally?

I don't think there are many of us who escape all fear and worry surrounding childbirth; the best most people can do is control it to some level. As no one can ever promise perfect issue-free outcomes in birth, it's not possible to have complete reassurance and peace. That said, if you can control the anxiety, I promise you, you can have a wonderful birth experience and enjoy every minute.

As a counsellor, I was acutely aware that lying to myself about my fear of the birth was not an option. I also understood that not allowing myself to think certain worries would only magnify the fear. So with this in mind I gave myself full permission to think about and process my fears surrounding the birth of my daughters.

I was careful about the language I chose to use around my births. If people asked me, 'Are you nervous?' I would answer, 'I am so excited to meet my baby.' I believe this helped prepare my brain for a positive experience.

My first epic fear was, what if we don't bring our baby home from the hospital? Even voicing that fear was hard, to be honest, as I was almost too scared to say it out loud. But as soon as I did, I felt relief. Andy and I talked about my anxiety, and he wisely said, 'Zoë, if we bring home an empty car seat, then we will find a way to cope, and we will survive.' Did this remove the fear? No, of course it didn't, but it felt good to talk about the terror I was carrying, and simply by verbalising it, it helped me emotionally.

My second fear was, what if something went wrong in the deliveries? I asked my consultant to explain all eventualities to me so that my imagination didn't have to make up potential scenarios. Again, this helped me no end as, just by voicing my concerns, I removed a little of the anxiety.

The week before my daughters were due to be delivered, I tried to view this time as similar to the week before a vacation. I spent time packing cases for us, and thinking of lots of nice things we could take with us to the hospital. I treated myself and got my nails and toes professionally manicured. I got my hair done, and did face masks and other beauty treatments. Every time a wave of panic went over me, I told myself this was due to the excitement of meeting my child. We also spent lots of quality time with family and friends, and this really helped keep me occupied.

On the days my girls were being born, I focused on staying present. I made sure I felt supported and also in control. I knew my choices would be listened to, and I felt secure with the medical team around me.

What followed with both births was truly beautiful. I would happily relive them over and over again. I hope you have a happy and positive birthing experience and find as much joy in the delivery as I did.

Today I am grateful for

DAY 2

Task

What do you hope the birth of your baby will be like? Once you have written your vision of the birth you hope for, try to hold on to this every time you think of the delivery.

Today I am grateful for

DAY 3

Daisy's Story

Nothing prepares you for those heartbreaking words, 'I'm sorry, but there is no heartbeat.' This wasn't our first loss, so something inside me felt like I should have been more prepared, that somehow I should have been stronger and handled it better this time. Except this time, it felt worse.

This time we had made it further than ever before, and were only two days away from our first scan. I hadn't felt right for a few days, but I continued as normal. For weeks, I had looked out for every sign that our baby had died. I visited the bathroom more times than I needed just to 'check'. I endlessly googled symptoms that I should or shouldn't be feeling for how many weeks I was. Anything to give me hope that this pregnancy wasn't going to end in the same way that our first had. But there was nothing, no sign. I felt sick, I was incredibly tired, and my stomach was growing. So when I visited the bathroom for the millionth time on that particular day and noticed that I was bleeding, my heart didn't just sink, it plummeted. Why now? I was so close. My husband and I tried to remain hopeful while we sat in A&E for what felt like hours, but then the news came. Except they said that they couldn't be

100 per cent sure and I would need to come back the following day for another internal scan to confirm their suspicions. I went home to put our children to bed, and as I looked at them, I remember feeling such guilt and sadness. They didn't know it yet, but I had news that would crush their dreams of another sibling. I held them tighter than I ever had before.

I felt all sorts of emotions that evening – deep sadness, anger (why *again*?), disappointment, guilt. I even felt some sort of relief that the three months of not knowing was over, for which I later felt so guilty.

Once the doctors had confirmed that our baby had died, the weeks that followed were gruelling. Labour, surgery, pain, funeral planning. Life had been taken from us too early, and I was grieving not having had the opportunity to introduce this baby to my other children, and not having the opportunity to be a parent again.

Looking back now, the months that followed were incredibly painful. My husband and I quickly decided that we wouldn't try again. We couldn't bear the pain, and anyway our family was probably complete after all. I quickly visited the doctor and settled on some contraception; I got a new job, and life was taking a different turn. What I see now, though, is that these were heat-of-the-moment decisions that only enhanced the numbness that I felt. I rushed into a new life that didn't involve pregnancy conversations or anything that would keep me lingering on what had just happened. I made a lot of mistakes in those following months and didn't allow myself the time that I really needed to heal. Months later, when my husband and I discovered that we were both considering 'trying' again, it felt like a shock but also a very peaceful confirmation that the decision we made days after the miscarriage wasn't the right one.

Pregnancy post-loss is hard; it's a kaleidoscope of emotions. Hope, joy, fear, expectation, excitement, guilt and renewed grief. It deserves greater understanding and recognition, as I discovered both the first time and initially in this pregnancy. What follows the storm, though, is truly beautiful. To hold your baby for the first time, watching their chest rise and fall, seeing their little mouth making those sucking movements and to hear that initial cry is like nothing else. No matter what we had been through in those early days, this day trumped it all. And now again, as I write this, I am five months pregnant; I couldn't be more excited for another baby to join our family. Yes, it's sometimes scary too – and I've learnt not to feel bad about that fear, it's only natural – but mostly this pregnancy is full of new adventure, new dreams and waiting for that next little kick to come!

Today I am grateful for

DAY 4

Support – Bringing your baby home

It can be hard to imagine ever bringing your baby home following baby loss, but I encourage you to try to imagine it, as in a few weeks you will be doing just that.

The day we brought both our girls home was utterly beautiful and very surreal.

Esmé was the first little one we brought home. As I had had a C-section, movement wasn't super-easy for me, but the pain was totally manageable, and nothing took away an ounce of the joy of putting our little girl in her car seat and walking out of the hospital. The journey home was exciting and terrifying; I noticed every driver who wasn't following the Highway Code! Having walked in our door so many times with empty arms, I can't even truly explain the moment we got to walk in holding Esmé. Let me add here that none of our joy negated or erased an ounce of the pain, but having experienced the pain, we truly valued this feeling of joy and happiness.

My parents came and stayed with us, which enabled Andy and me to have periods of sleep throughout the night (as it turned out we only make children who don't need sleep!). I loved those first weeks, though don't get me wrong, they were also SO hard. Chronic sleep deprivation was a new thing for me, and I quickly learnt why it's used as a torture technique, but I really did feel a joy that I had never felt before. I was getting to raise a child, something I had dreamt of, longed for and, for a while, never thought would happen.

It took us about three to four weeks to get into a great routine, and for our bodies to adapt to the lack of sleep.

The one thing that shocked me was that the worry I had when I was pregnant continued. Instead of being worried about Esmé being delivered safely, I was now worried about her catching viruses or germs from visitors. I was also worried about cot death. It took real work to stop this worry, and in hindsight, I wished I had worked harder at stopping and controlling the fear while I was pregnant, by doing mindfulness exercises and talking about my underlying fears, which could have released me from their power. But even with having to navigate the worry . . . I LOVED, LOVED, LOVED being a mum.

I am now the mother of an 11-year-old and an eight-year-old, and I can honestly say that the joy has never left me.

Being a parent is a true honour, and I hope you love it as much as I do.

Here are six things I wish I had been told as a new parent:

1. A lot of babies get jaundice, and most of the time it goes away without treatment. Both of mine got it, and it scared me a lot – now I know I didn't need to panic at all.
2. When you are told sleep when your baby sleeps, it's TRUE! Do it, don't question it. Try not to view time as day and night, view each day as 24 hours. If your baby sleeps for five hours from 11am to 4pm, you sleep then too, even though it's daytime. You need your rest. Once your baby is in a routine, you can focus on getting back to day and night again.
3. Don't be afraid to lock your doors and say no to visitors. The first seven to 10 days are all about you and your little one. If you want to stay in your PJs, then do it. Eat lovely food, have all your favourite films ready to play (even if that's at 3am) and try to have enough babygrows in a drawer so that you don't need to be doing laundry every day.
4. Tiredness can make even the most patient and kind person grouchy and irritable. Be mindful of this with yourself and your partner, and be quick to forgive, and first to apologise.
5. Make sure you get on with your GP and health visitor and, if you don't, ask to move to another. It's really important as a parent that you feel heard and have people around you who listen to concerns and are also good at bringing reassurance.
6. Listen to your gut – it's called mum instinct for a reason. You are wired to know when something may be wrong with your baby. Yes, fear can make you panic and confuse this instinct, but if you are worried, that is a valid enough reason to get your child checked, and you should always be listened to.

Today I am grateful for

DAY 5

Journalling your pregnancy

What gestation is your baby today? _____

How big are they? _____

What symptoms are you now feeling?

What do you want to remember about how you are feeling or what you are experiencing?

> I refused to let grief define me,
> I chose to let it refine me instead.

ZOË CLARK-COATES

Today I am grateful for

DAY 6

Support – Your relationship with your partner

Having a child will change every relationship in your life, and that includes the one with your partner. Suddenly you have a third little person in your home, a person who is highly demanding and would like to captivate you 24 hours a day. Some find the relationship with their spouse gets even stronger, but for others having a child can be a real strain on a relationship. So what are my top tips?

1. Make as much time as possible for each other. I don't necessarily mean establishing date nights in those early days; what is more important is to keep being interested in each other. Make sure you ask how each other's day has been, and listen to the reply. Talk about struggles you may be having and try to deal with those as a couple. It's so easy for the complete focus to be on the baby, and that can be detrimental to a relationship.

2. Try to work together to cope with disturbed sleep by taking it in turns to look after the baby so that the other

can sleep. Humans need rest and, by working together, you may be able to give each other a few undisturbed hours.
3. Many people find themselves arguing a lot more with their spouse after having children. Maybe this is because of increased stress levels, but I also think it's because you suddenly have a lot more subjects or issues to disagree on or be irritated by. Keeping the lines of communication open is vital and trying to be as patient as possible can help a huge amount.

Early on in our marriage Andy and I established some ground rules that we are still grateful for today. These are:

1. Never walk out of a room when arguing or angry – we committed always to resolve whatever the issue is.
2. If one of us brings an issue to the table the other can't say, 'Well, I did that because you did this.' We agreed that if an issue wasn't important enough to bring up at the time, it shouldn't then be used as a weapon later. I promise you this decision is a game-changer. It means you don't hold on to resentment or grudges. You have to decide in the moment, 'Do I care enough about how he just spoke to me to discuss it?' If I decide no, then it's dropped and never brought up.
3. The third and final thing is we don't ever say anything like, 'As I have already said' in any discussion. We agreed this makes the other party feel bad for asking again, or stupid for not hearing it the first time, and it causes bad feeling. If someone says, 'I need to hear you say sorry', it doesn't help to hear, 'I have already said that to you.' If they are asking for an apology, it means they haven't 'heard it', they haven't 'felt it', so it needs to be repeated until it is felt, heard and accepted.

These three ground rules have been so helpful to us, and I hope by sharing them, they may be useful to you too.

Today I am grateful for

DAY 7

Journal

What could you do to help make your relationship with your partner (or family and friends if you don't have a partner) stronger and healthier?

When people tell me 'I used to be happy'
it breaks my heart.

Whatever pain one has gone through,
or trauma one has faced,
happiness remains accessible
to those who want it.

We may, of course, find our happiness
in a very different place than before.
It may no longer be found in the
eyes of someone we love . . .

We may now find it in the sunrise,
or in the service of others . . .

But it is always available to us all.

ZOË CLARK-COATES

Today I am grateful for

WEEK 38

· ·

DAY 1

Support – Grief layers

It is very common post-delivery to have new layers of grief surface. I am often emailed by new parents in an utter panic, fearing that they are suffering from postnatal depression, when actually what they are encountering is another grief layer being processed. So how can you tell what is grief and what is postnatal depression? It can be tricky for people to identify what is grief and a natural hormone shift, and what is postnatal depression, so please speak with your doctor or midwife and get a formal assessment. They will ask you questions and possibly ask you to fill in a survey, after which they should be able to diagnose you.

How does one handle a grief layer surfacing, while also looking after a newborn?

Firstly, please don't be scared. Understand that as grief is a lifelong journey, any event can bring up a new grief layer at any point in your life, and it's natural that having another child should do this.

My best advice for handling the emergence of more grief is to talk about it. Tell your partner or family and friends what you are feeling. Just the pure act of talking can help you move through the fresh feelings of grief that have surfaced. If talking doesn't help, I would suggest one of two things. You will find help and support in my earlier book *The Baby Loss Guide* to help you gently process your emotions.

Secondly, I encourage you to get professional help. That may mean reaching out to a charity such as sayinggoodbye.org, or it may mean finding a counsellor or speaking with your

GP and asking for therapy. The vital thing is you are dealing with the feelings that you are experiencing. If you shove your feelings down, they will pop up at a later date, so it is much better to deal with them as they emerge.

Today I am grateful for

DAY 2

Task

Write down all of the emotions you are currently feeling. The stronger the emotion, the bigger you should write. So are you feeling . . . Happy? Sad? Optimistic? Nervous? Joyful? Fill this box with words.

Today I am grateful for

(blank box)

DAY 3

Today I am sharing the answers to five questions that I am regularly asked as CEO of The Mariposa Trust (sayinggoodbye.org), by people who are facing pregnancy after loss.

1. What was the hardest issue you found in pregnancy?

For me, the hardest issues were the physical symptoms, especially in my pregnancy with Brontë, as I was very poorly until I delivered her. The other issue was the daily battle with my mind to believe all was well. It is only when you have delivered your child that you realise how much mental energy that has taken from you.

2. What helped you survive the nine months of pregnancy?

Keeping as busy as I was physically able to be. I found distraction was my friend, and the more I could think of other things that were not pregnancy-related, the better I felt emotionally.

3. How did you get a good night's sleep?

I didn't, to be honest, but some things helped me.

I slept with a lot of pillows, and this helped my back and my hips. I also slept with a pillow in between my legs, and this really helped the pain in my hips.

I decided to use the loo at night in the dark (or in very dim light), as then I couldn't check if I could see red. Anyone who has suffered from blood loss fear will understand that using the loo after a previous loss can be super-scary. The moment your adrenaline starts running it can be so hard to go back to sleep, so I chose not to check for blood at night, and I tried to keep myself calm and half asleep when using the loo for my constant bathroom visits at night.

I made sure my sheets were 100 per cent cotton, and I would only wear cotton clothing at night, so my temperature was more stable.

I had things on standby to listen to if I needed to be soothed back to sleep – you may want to have music or podcasts lined up. Sometimes listening to a distracting programme helps people get to sleep quicker, as it stops your brain trying to process fears or worries.

4. Did you want more children?

As my pregnancy with Brontë was so scary, and my life was literally 'in the balance' for some time, I didn't feel I even had the choice to have more children, to be honest. As soon as she arrived and was safe, it just felt like the right thing to say was OK, we are done. If I had had a smooth and easy pregnancy with her, perhaps we would have chosen to have more children, but we didn't, and my priority was to make sure my daughters had a mother to raise them.

5. Do you struggle with knowing that the children you have here with you are only here due to the children who died?

I don't actually, but I entirely understand why so many people struggle with this. Yes, it's true, if my first three children hadn't died, Esmé would not be here now. Likewise, if Samuel hadn't died, Brontë wouldn't be here now, but they did die, and Esmé and Brontë lived. I will never be OK with my five babies dying, and I don't have to be. I will never understand why they died, but I have now found a sense of peace in not knowing why they did. All I know is this – I love every one of my children, those who are here, and those who have gone ahead. I will never understand why some children need to run ahead before others can arrive, but that is OK, I don't need to understand it. I don't need to have all the answers, and I don't need to feel any guilt about embracing the children I am blessed to raise. As humans we are conditioned by society to question everything, to strive for answers and to try to make sense of every confusing situation, but I really believe we can waste a lot of our lives doing this, and it also comes with a huge sacrifice, and that is the sacrifice of our peace.

Today I am grateful for

DAY 4

Support – Being kind to yourself

Once your little one is in your arms, you will probably find yourself thinking of yourself last; I know I did. Suddenly your needs and desires don't seem important anymore, compared to the needs and desires of your child. While I believe this is part of how we are created as mothers, I also feel we need to be wise to ensure we do consider ourselves a priority. Your physical health matters. Your mental health matters. Your happiness and peace matter. By looking after yourself, you are also ultimately doing right by your child, as they will flourish if you are happy and content.

Mum guilt is a real thing, and something you will quickly become accustomed to feeling. As the guilt gets a louder and louder voice, it can be hard to ignore, and then we start to put ourselves last. I advise you to be super-mindful of this tendency to deprioritise yourself, and try to consider situations rationally. You do not need to feel guilty for taking time to sleep, bathe, exercise, read or engage in activities that make you calmer, happier or more healthy – please remember this! It can even help to make yourself a sign reminding yourself that you matter too, and stick it on your bathroom door to read often.

Today I am grateful for

DAY 5

Journalling your pregnancy

What gestation is your baby today? _____

How big are they? _____

What symptoms are you now feeling?

What do you want to remember about how you are feeling or what you are experiencing?

Sometimes people fear falling,
but it makes the world of difference
if you know there is someone
waiting to catch you.

ZOË CLARK-COATES

Today I am grateful for

DAY 6

Support – Impending sadness at not being pregnant anymore

Some of you may laugh at this, as you can't wait for your pregnancy to be over, while others will be nodding 'yes'. If you have spent a long time trying to get pregnant, or longing to be pregnant, it can be hard imagining that in a few weeks you will no longer be carrying your little one in your body. For months and months, you have been the only one who has helped them survive, and only you have carried them within since the moment they were conceived. So it's a big transition when they are born, as you will probably then be sharing them with others.

I really missed my pregnancy bump. I missed knowing my baby automatically went everywhere with me, but the sensations I missed were tiny compared to what I gained once they arrived in my arms.

I dealt with my feelings of sadness about the end of pregnancy by focusing on gratitude that I had a child to raise. Every time a wave of upset hit me, I counteracted it with a list of things I was so happy about. I also reminded myself of the not-so-nice parts of being pregnant.

Be prepared for a mixture of varying and random feelings to hit you post-delivery. Some will make complete sense; others won't. Hormones, a lack of sleep, huge emotional upheaval are all responsible for these feelings trying to take up residence in your head. Not all of them need to be processed; some can just be acknowledged as being present, and then you let them fade away. Other feelings may need talking about to help you process them.

Today I am grateful for

DAY 7

Journal

How would you describe your pregnancy? What do you want to remember most about it?

One of the things I am asked the most is
how do you support someone you love
through grief and fear?

People often think I will give them this complex
map to navigate, with a list of rules to follow,
but they couldn't be more wrong.

There is only one thing everyone needs to do,
and that is to 'show up'.

Show up even if you don't know what to say.
Show up even if you are afraid to see
someone in terrible pain.
Show up even if you feel helpless,
scared and vulnerable.

I promise you however hard it is
for you to witness the suffering,
it is harder for them to carry the grief and worry.

However fearful you are of saying the wrong thing,
they are more terrified of facing this alone.

So show up even if you want to run for the hills,
even if you stumble on your words,
even if you say nothing at all.

Just be present, hold their hand,
and I promise you, you will have made a difference
because you have shown up.

ZOË CLARK-COATES

Today I am grateful for

WEEK 39

DAY 1

Support – Post-traumatic growth

We hear often about post-traumatic stress, but we hear little, if anything, about post-traumatic growth. You may never have come across this term as it is not commonly discussed. Post-traumatic growth is described as a positive psychological change arising from adversity, which ultimately creates a higher level of functioning. By adapting to challenges, and by changing their understanding of the world and their place in it, individuals with post-traumatic growth develop life-changing psychological shifts that can be deeply meaningful. To put it simply: the trauma you have lived through can propel you to a new level of joy or a greater sense of purpose in life.

I am a big believer in PTG and believe this is why I now feel more joy than I ever felt before encountering loss, and why I find a greater meaning to life than ever before.

I can often be heard saying that my losses carved out huge valleys in my soul, but these valleys have now been filled with joy. I longed to be able to talk about my five children who ran ahead with a smile on my face, I didn't want them only to be remembered with tears, and I worked hard to get to that place. You may also desire this, and yet it may feel impossible to achieve, but I can assure you that with help, time and work it is within your reach.

Today I am grateful for

DAY 2

Task

How do you want the baby (or babies) you have lost to be remembered? Also, how do you want to feel when you talk about them?

Today I am grateful for

DAY 3

Amy's Story

A few years ago, my twin girls, Charlotte and Esme, were born at 26 weeks' gestation. We heartbreakingly lost Esme at seven weeks old, due to extreme prematurity, septicaemia and ventriculitis. Charlotte continued her fight and got stronger by the day. She came home on her due date, exactly three months later.

I spent my days mothering Charlotte and nights grieving for Esme. Five months after losing Esme, I struggled. My smiles felt forced, and the days became darker. I self-referred for bereavement counselling. This was the hardest phone call and the first time that I said Esme's full name out loud since she had died. Those next six months of counselling were invaluable and enabled me to move forward and begin to understand my grief.

I had felt broody ever since the girls were born. I wasn't sure if this was because I had had a premature birth and was desperate to experience and prove to myself and others that I could carry a baby to full term, whether it was because I had lost a baby, or whether I just enjoyed motherhood and naturally wanted another baby. I became obsessed with looking out for siblings similar in age. I would ask mums how old their eldest was when they started trying for a second. I desperately sought reassurance that it was perfectly normal to want another child and not a result of prematurity or loss of a baby.

Although my second pregnancy was mentally one of my toughest challenges, it healed me in many ways and allowed me to accept and love my body.

Seeing full-term bumps and attending baby showers became easier and I was able to forgive my harsh thoughts of self-blame for the girls' prematurity and Esme's death. Looking back, it makes me feel sad; I felt ashamed and embarrassed. I saw my body as weak and incapable of carrying my babies to full term.

We were advised by our consultant to wait at least a year before trying again. When Charlotte was 15 months old, I fell pregnant.

At eight weeks pregnant, I met my consultants and had a scan to find out if it was multiple pregnancies. It took a while to digest that I was carrying one baby as I still wanted that chance to carry twins to full term.

Our appointments with the consultants helped us to piece together and provide closure as to why Charlotte's (Twin 1) waters went at 24 weeks. I felt confident enough to confide my biggest anxieties and fears with them. Their reassurance, professionalism and empathy provided instant relief, and they played a huge role in supporting us through the toughest of times.

The majority of my pregnancy was spent in survival mode. I held my breath every time I went to the toilet and breathed a sigh of relief when I saw no blood. Living by the day was all I could do, to manage my thoughts, anxieties and fears.

By 18 weeks pregnant, I turned into a frantic knitter and knitted hats for family and friends. It gave me something to focus on and helped prevent my mind from thinking intrusive thoughts.

One of my best decisions was returning to my favourite aqua-natal class at 20 weeks pregnant. It took courage to go. I was nervous about seeing someone pregnant with twins and scared of flashbacks, remembering the excitement about having twins. These classes were great therapy, and by talking about my pregnancies and my loss, I found I had many fond memories of my twin pregnancy. That's not to say I didn't have a good cry in the pool as I painfully remembered what could have been. A lady pregnant with twins attended. Yes, it hurt but I was able to have empathy with her, knowing how it felt. It was much harder to live with the fear of what could happen than what had actually happened.

The most challenging time was from 22 weeks to 27 weeks. This period included coping with the anxieties leading up to Twin 1's waters going at 24 weeks and the girls being born at 26 weeks and six days. Despite only being pregnant with one baby, I found it difficult to separate my two pregnancies.

Just like any other day of my pregnancy, those anxious days came and went and were just 'normal' days. As I reached the third trimester, these 'normal' days, where everything just ticked by, encouraged my feelings of hope to grow stronger.

Every stage of my pregnancy brought with it new anxieties: miscarriage, prematurity and then stillbirth. However, it was during my final trimester that I allowed myself to begin to imagine that this baby might be coming home.

After 27 weeks pregnant, there were more occasions when I imagined Charlotte playing with her sibling, and I found the courage to sort through her baby clothes. I managed to bring a bag of second-hand baby clothes through the front door, something I had been unable to do for the past 10 weeks. These moments felt like a weight had been lifted and the feelings of happiness and hope started to outweigh those of fear.

My final milestone to overcome in my pregnancy was reaching the point at which we lost Esme. If I'd remained pregnant, she would have been 35+1 weeks' gestation. However, by that point in Esme's life, I'd already had seven weeks of getting to know her and dreaming of the day we would come home. I found coping with the power of pregnancy hormones tricky enough, but when coupled with trauma and grief, I often found it confusing to decipher what and how I was feeling.

My husband really struggled with bonding with my bump and rarely touched it. He didn't like touching it. I found this really tough, and on many occasions, it made me feel alone. This upset me. He was, however, an incredible support emotionally. He was there for me every time I worried about baby's movements and gave me that gentle encouragement to get in the car and get checked out. He always knew exactly how to comfort and reassure me and said just what I needed to hear to understand that my anxieties were perfectly normal.

As hope grew, I felt desperate to experience everything I had grieved and had been robbed of: packing my hospital bag, my waters breaking, the frantic drive to the hospital, experiencing the sensation of contractions and, above all, giving birth vaginally and immediately holding my baby. I wanted these so badly. These hopes remained in my subconscious. I was frightened of allowing myself to think, dream and imagine them, for fear of everything being ripped away from me.

I started an online hypnobirthing course and found this very useful. Everything became a little more real and exciting.

I was induced on a Saturday night and went into labour early Sunday morning. Due to the nature of the induction process, I had an epidural. I spent the next four hours pain-free but could feel my body and my baby working together. I felt safe, happy and excited.

My husband Connor and I proudly spoke about Charlotte and Esme and our time on the neonatal unit. I felt like I had known my midwife forever and she helped make that day such a joyful experience.

Archibald James Campbell was born on 10 June at 2.47pm, weighing 8lb 7oz. Six days late.

It was one of the happiest days of my life, and I spent it in a bubble of love. I was relaxed and in this surreal, worry-free and euphoric place.

He was everything I had dreamt of and more.

Today I am grateful for

DAY 4

Support – Telling children about siblings who have died

I am constantly asked, 'How do I tell my children about the babies that I have lost?'

I believe that children can handle virtually all information, it just has to be said to them in the right way, and in words that they understand. Of course, they may not truly comprehend or understand what certain things mean until they mature, but I would encourage you to share your family's truth with them from day one.

I never wanted the children we lost to be a secret; I wanted everyone to always feel totally comfortable with talking about them with me, and around my family. This meant we had to be open about what happened from the start. Because we always spoke about the five babies who went ahead of us, we never needed to have a big discussion with the girls, they were just always aware that they had sisters and a brother who weren't here with us.

Of course, over the years they have asked questions, and when they have, we have honestly answered them. Because of this openness, they will happily talk about life and loss without any fear or upset. To them, it's the same as talking about any other life event.

My advice is to not be afraid to talk about death and loss with children; they are extremely adaptable and capable of handling it.

Saying Goodbye have got an incredible short video on their website, which explains baby loss in a really simple way to children, so if you have been seeking a practical resource such as this, head to:
www.sayinggoodbye.org/information/children

Today I am grateful for

DAY 5

Journalling your pregnancy

What gestation is your baby today? _____

How big are they? _____

What symptoms are you now feeling?

What do you want to remember about how you are feeling or what you are experiencing?

. . . .

The aftershocks of grief are far-reaching;
this is perhaps one of the most
unrecognised parts of loss.

. . . . ZOË CLARK-COATES . . . .

Today I am grateful for

DAY 6

Support – Body image

Pregnancy, childbirth and breastfeeding can radically change your body. For some, these changes feel hard to bear, while for others, they are easy to accept and gratefully received.

I personally didn't mind the changes – I saw stretch marks as reminders that I had been blessed to carry a child. I saw my C-section scar as my gold medal for crossing the finishing line. But what should you do if you do struggle with scars, a changed shape, or if you weigh more than you would like?

The first step is to give yourself time to adjust to the inevitable physical changes post-pregnancy; some of these changes may only be temporary, while others may be permanent. Give yourself time for those temporary changes to adjust, and give yourself space to come to terms with your new body. Be kind to yourself and try not to judge your body harshly. Only with time can you determine whether you want to do something about those physical changes or not, such as joining a gym. But make sure any steps you take are made out of love for your body, and not out of punishment.

Please remember that your body has achieved something magnificent and deserves to be celebrated.

Today I am grateful for

DAY 7

Journal

What changes in your body or your mind do you appreciate?

Though the seasons change,
my love will forever remain.

ZOË CLARK-COATES

Today I am grateful for

WEEK 40

• •

DAY 1

Support – You've nearly made it over the finish line

You are nearly there, you have run the race and are nearly over that finish line. If you found out you were pregnant very early on, I imagine you feel like you have been pregnant for an extremely long time.

The important thing now is to try to relax as much as possible and stay present. This is when anxiety can start to take over, and just remaining focused and consciously choosing to think positively can help.

If you have any worries at all, please get them out in the open and don't panic alone. Call your midwife or hospital and ask them any questions you may have. Importantly, always get monitored if you feel any decrease or increase in your baby's movements, and please don't feel like you are wasting anyone's time even if you do this every single day. The only important thing now is your baby arriving safely in your arms!

Today I am grateful for

DAY 2

Task

Write a letter to your child that they can read on their 18th birthday.

Dear

Today I am grateful for

Nicky's Story

I remember the day I found out I was pregnant again like it's etched permanently in my mind and heart. It was the first few days of the new year, and we (my husband and daughter and I) were on holiday in New Zealand. I was seven days late for my period and I never even considered I would be pregnant. And that is really true because I had quite a few rum cocktails on New Year's Eve! I just thought my body was a bit out of whack because of all the travelling, and my period would come once we'd settled into our new environment.

But something that morning felt different – I'd recovered from my New Year's Eve hangover but was still feeling super-bloated and off. And then the thought popped into my mind, but I barely allowed myself to think it: 'Maybe I'm pregnant!' Followed by an immediate shutdown: 'Can I allow myself to even think it? I can't bear the disappointment if I'm not. And what if I am and then I lose it again?' My mind was racing as I tried to breathe and compose myself.

Over the previous three years, I had lost two babies. Both utterly and completely crushed me. Both brought on so much grief; I wondered if I'd ever get through it. I never in my wildest dreams imagined it would be so hard and painful to try to have a second baby. Conceiving Teia (our daughter) was so easy, so straightforward that I totally took it for granted that I could just 'have another'. But then it turned into this utter nightmare. Each time I got pregnant my babies didn't survive. The second time the loss was so traumatic, physically and emotionally, as I haemorrhaged and lost an enormous amount of blood. I suffered from post-traumatic shock for a year. After that, something in me and my heart died with my baby. I gave up. I didn't even dare to want another. I could barely let my husband touch me again for nearly half a year as I was so scared of getting pregnant again.

So as I sat on the bed, bloated stomach, seven days late, mind racing, I was overcome with complete terror and utter excitement at exactly the same time. I decided to go for a walk on my own into town to get a pregnancy test, but I didn't want anyone to know. I kept it a secret from everyone, even my husband, telling them I just wanted a bit of time alone. I remember I couldn't even really allow myself to think it, almost as though if I said it out loud then it would be real, and I would care and then it would crush me if I lost it again.

So in my frozen state, barely even daring to breathe, I walked into the pharmacy and bought a test. As I sat in the public toilet waiting for the line, something in me just knew. I'm not sure how, I'm not sure why, but I knew it was going to tell me I was pregnant. And there it was – a strong, bold pink line, undeniably showing me that once again I had a beautiful baby growing within me.

I felt so happy, so happy there are no words to describe it fully. Something in my heart burst open as I let it all in and realised all along I had wanted this but didn't dare let myself, and I burst into tears, crying with joy and fear all at the same time.

The first trimester was tricky. Even though somehow I just knew this one was meant to reside earthside, I couldn't trust anything anymore. So I insisted on paying a fortune for private scans. The NHS were amazing, so supportive, and gave me extra scans whenever I asked, which I'm extremely grateful for. Each scan showed us that this little one was strong, healthy and not looking like he was going anywhere.

Still, I didn't fully let myself get complacent.

Once I moved into my second trimester, I tried to relax a little. Now I look back on it I can understand why I barely exercised and I also ate a lot more. I was so scared to take any risks, so scared to do anything that would cause damage and I comfort-ate to ease the anxiety. But I realise now I didn't share about what I was feeling with anyone. Almost as though if I even said my fears out loud, it would make something happen, so I kept it all inside and pretended it wasn't there.

Alongside all of this, I was so grateful. I spent so much time talking to my son inside of me, rubbing my belly, holding my belly. Once I could feel him kicking, I felt many moments of pure and utter joy every single day.

Once I was in my third trimester, and we started the process of preparing for birth, again without my really being aware of it at the time, the fear started coming back. I was planning for a home birth, but I was willing to do anything just to make sure he got out safely. In the final weeks before he arrived, I stopped being able to sleep. I had heard some very sad news that a friend of mine had lost her baby, and as soon as I heard that, I could no longer sleep. Every night, my husband and daughter fast asleep, I would sit upstairs on the sofa, watching movies until 3am, eating crisps and comfort food. I had no awareness that the reason I was doing that was because I was so scared to lose my son. I could barely sit with myself. Once again I couldn't say my fears out loud in case they became real, so I buried them deep down and didn't sleep and ate to get through it.

I went into labour four days past my due date.

Strangely I was so grateful for every single contraction. Every one of them was bringing my boy closer to me. After 27 hours of intense, strong contractions and enormous nausea, I was losing so much energy that we went into hospital to have some pain relief. But once we got there my waters broke, and there were a few complications, and I was told I needed a C-section. I remember being so exhausted and thinking that I honestly didn't care anymore about the perfect birth, I just wanted him in my arms. Nothing was going to get in the way of me holding my son this time.

At 12.15am on 8 September, my beautiful boy, Calum, was born. Weighing a whopping 10lb, the doctor pulled him out of me and placed him on my chest. I couldn't believe how beautiful, how perfect, how utterly amazing he was. Both my husband and I cried with such gratitude, overcome with love and joy.

I promise you, every single day since the day he was born, I look at him and feel overwhelmingly grateful. He is an absolute gift and a blessing. He is my miracle baby. The one I never thought I would be able to have. The one I almost gave up on. Every now and then, when I'm holding him, I whisper in his ear and tell him that secretly, deep down buried in my heart, I never ever fully gave up, that I always wished and prayed for him.

Today I am grateful for

DAY 4

Support – Acknowledging good or bad care

I want to encourage you to write to anyone and everyone who has offered you good or poor care in this pregnancy. The reason I suggest doing it now is once your little one arrives in your arms, you will have little time to do this and it often then never gets done. We can only change the poor care that's offered by pointing out when it's happening. Likewise, we should be rewarding the good care so that it can be increased and commended. So take some time today to write to GPs, midwives, hospitals etc. and together we can make sure all care in the future is first class.

Today I am grateful for

DAY 5

Journalling your pregnancy

What gestation is your baby today? _____

How big are they? _____

What symptoms are you now feeling?

What do you want to remember about how you are feeling or what you are experiencing?

Grief is never comfortable;
it is always agony.

It is the equivalent of crawling on your
knees through a burning forest,
yet the world often acts like
it's a stroll in the park.

• • • • • • • • • • • • ZOË CLARK-COATES • • • • • • • • • • • • •

Today I am grateful for

DAY 6

Support – Celebrating yourself

Pregnancy after loss is both beautiful and hard. It is like walking a tightrope with no training, and no crash mat beneath. At times you may have felt you are preparing yourself emotionally for more loss, rather than eagerly awaiting new life. You will have learnt that most people seem to think positive thinking is the answer to everything, but mamas who have gone through loss know better than that. At times we are powerless, and that is perhaps what is most scary. Our children are our heartbeat, and when we have to accept that there is only so much we can do to protect them, it's a very bitter pill to swallow. BUT you are nearly there, my friend. I want to honour you, and want you to celebrate you too. Women seem conditioned to undervalue their achievements, to minimise their accomplishments, and we most certainly do this when it comes to pregnancy. Today take time to look at what you have done. See how far you have travelled. Consider the hurdles you have had to jump. And then . . . say to yourself, 'Well done, I made it through.'

Today I am grateful for

DAY 7

Journal

What do you want to remember about this pregnancy? Use this space to record anything you want never to forget.

No baby can ever replace another;
every single baby is unique and precious.

Any child who is born following a baby who has died is not a replacement; they are a longed-for sibling and a gift to their family.

ZOË CLARK-COATES

Today I am grateful for

CONCLUSION

Soon you will have a sibling to the child you have lost in your arms. In a perfect world, you would have every child you have created and loved in your arms, and I am so sorry that so many of us have to live with some of our children missing.

I want to tell you how proud I am of you. There were times back there when I am sure you doubted you had the strength to make it through, but you have done it.

By facing your fears you have gained resilience and strength. By teaching yourself to manage your stress responses you have overcome situations that felt incomprehensible.

You have learnt things over the past 40 weeks that will make you a better mother, a better partner, a better friend, a better person.

You are about to cross that longed-for finish line, and I am sure it feels surreal.

Loss changes you forever, but so does pregnancy and so does having the opportunity to raise a longed-for baby, so I hope you enjoy this next chapter of your life.

I'd like to think that this book has been a friend to you, and that the words within it have helped you navigate your pregnancy. I also hope it taught you tools and techniques that can be used throughout your life whenever you face challenges.

Please come find me on social media or get in touch (*see below*). I would love to share in your joy, see photos of your babies and hear your stories.

Remember, you are a warrior mum.

You are not defined by loss, but changed by loss, and now you get to teach your little one how to conquer this world.

Instagram – @Zoeadelle   Twitter – @ClarkCoates
Facebook – @ZoeAdelleCC   Pinterest – /zoeclarkcoates/
Website – www.zoeadelle.co.uk

Help and Resources

International support following baby loss and pregnancy after loss

Advice, support, befriending, international remembrance services, counselling, support via social media and more.

The Mariposa Trust – Saying Goodbye is the primary division which offers support post-baby loss, but the charity has many other divisions too.
- mariposatrust.org
- sayinggoodbye.org

The **GrowingYou** division supports people through pregnancy after loss.
- www.growingyou.org

Marriage counselling and support

- relate.org.uk
- themarriagecourses.org/try/the-marriage-course/

Bereavement support and counselling

- mariposatrust.org
- soultears.org
- sayinggoodbye.org
- psychotherapy.org.uk/find-a-therapist/

- cruse.org.uk
- childbereavementuk.org
- mind.org.uk
- nhs.uk/conditions/counselling/
- bacp.co.uk/search/Therapists
- acc-uk.org
- anxietyuk.org.uk
- counselling-directory.org.uk
- mindandsoulfoundation.org

Emotional support for people in distress

- Samaritans – samaritans.org
- SOBS – uksobs.org

Pre- and postnatal depression

- pandasfoundation.org.uk
- nct.org.uk

Thank You

Firstly, I want to thank you for choosing to read this book.

Huge thanks to Sarah, Lindsay, Becky, Nicola, Becki, Jill, Gemma, Claire, Emily, Rachel, Zoë B, Esther, Anna, Tyne, Laura, Bex, Daisy, Amy, Nicky, who all kindly shared their stories for this book, in the hope it makes others feel less alone. For some of you, I know it was the first time you have shared your stories – I am so very grateful that you trusted me and my book to voice your words.

Thanks to experts Dr Jacque Gerrard MBE, Dr Jessica Farren, Siobhan Abrahams, Nichola Ludlam-Raine, Clare Bourne and Helen Clint for sharing their knowledge.

Thanks to my agent Jane Graham Maw and my editor Pippa Wright, and all who have helped make this book come to pass at Orion Spring. You believe in me and my work and a mere thank you doesn't seem sufficient, to be honest, but thank you – thank you for entrusting me with and for giving me this platform to write books and support more people.

Thanks to Professor Jacqueline Dunkley-Bent OBE for always believing in me and championing my work, your support means the world to me.

Thanks to the pregnant friends who read through this book ahead of it being published to ensure it was helpful . . . your beautiful encouragement truly helped me.

Thanks to Rachel Ervin for cheering me on, I love you dear friend, and appreciated you allowing me to use you as a sounding board.

Thanks to the team at The Mariposa Trust. I am so

grateful to each of you. The charity team are not just 'team', they are so much more than that; they are family. You are all my heroes, you give up so much of your time and dedicate so much of your life to helping others and it is only by us working together globally that we are able to support as many people as we do.

Thank you to my wonderful family (especially my mum and dad who work alongside us at the charity), you are not 'just' my parents, you are our best friends.

To my friends who believe in me even when I don't believe in myself, thank you. We laugh together and we cry together. We sit under blankets sharing stories, and we walk on beaches discussing our dreams . . . you bring sunshine to my life.

The biggest thank you to Andy, my soulmate, and my two daughters, Esmé Emilia and Brontë Jemima – you are my world. The journey I have written about is all of our stories, we walked it together, and there are no people I would rather experience life with than you. You bring joy to my days and hope to my future. Thank you for being the best humans I know; I will love you forever.

The final thank you goes to God, without you I wouldn't be standing today. When I couldn't walk you carried me. When I sat crying on the floor, I felt you weeping next to me. Through it all, you made me brave. I don't often talk about my faith in my books, but it is such an important part of who I am, and why I do what I do.

Legacy Scheme

If this book has helped you, would you consider purchasing copies to help others?

Maybe you would like to buy a couple of copies for friends or family who have lost a baby and are now pregnant, or perhaps you might like to purchase copies in bulk? Many people around the world have fundraised to enable them to buy hundreds of copies of my other books, in honour of the baby they have lost. They then donate these books to hospitals, clinics, GP practices, churches or support groups, so anyone who has lost a baby gets given a copy as soon as they have encountered loss. They even write a personal message to the bereaved family in each book.

I would love people to do this with *Pregnancy After Loss* too, so when people find out they are pregnant, their midwife could give them this book to help them navigate pregnancy. If you want to be part of making that happen, email us today.

For more information, email:
legacy@pregnancyafterloss.org

About the Author

Zoë Clark-Coates BCAh is an award-winning charity CEO, business leader, counsellor, conference speaker, author and TV show host. For over 20 years she has been a trailblazer within PR, events and the media.

Following the loss of five babies, she co-founded the charity The Mariposa Trust (widely known by the name of its primary support division, sayinggoodbye.org) with her husband Andy, enabling her to use her training as a counsellor on a daily basis.

As an innovative leader, she has steered the charity to become a leading support organisation in the UK and globally, providing support that reaches over 50,000 people each week.

As a gifted communicator, she has earned the respect of politicians, the government and many high-profile celebrities and influencers. Zoë's skill as a writer prompted Arianna Huffington to invite her to start writing for the *Huffington Post*, which created the perfect platform to reach a new audience.

She has her own TV talk show, *Soul Tears*, where she interviews celebrities and people of note about their journeys through loss. She is also a trusted expert and media commentator for many other programmes on the BBC, ITV and Channel 5.

Zoë was appointed by the Secretary of State for Health as co-chair of the National Pregnancy Loss Review. As co-chair, she is responsible for advising the government and Department of Health on how better support and clinical care can be offered.